THE
SUPERSTAR
BODY

REAL WORLD TECHNIQUES FOR ACHIEVING YOUR GOALS

NICK ALDIS

First published by Pitch Publishing, 2015

Pitch Publishing
A2 Yeoman Gate
Yeoman Way
Durrington
BN13 3QZ
www.pitchpublishing.co.uk

A CIP catalogue record is available for this book
from the British Library.

ISBN 978-1-90962-643-0

Typesetting and origination by Pitch Publishing

Printed in Malta by Melita Press

Contents

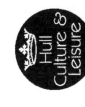

Tel: 01482 300 30

...ans.co.uk

with compliments

Central Library, Albion Street, Hull HU1 3TF

Tel: 01482   Fax: 01482

For my son,
Donovan Patrick Aldis.

Everything I do is to make
your life better.

Disclaimer and a little housekeeping...

My name is Nick Aldis. To some of you, I will be better known as the characters I have played on TV, like Magnus from TNA *Impact Wrestling* or Oblivion from *Gladiators*. But I'm also a magazine columnist, I've been lifting weights since I was 12, and I've dedicated my life to the pursuit of physical and mental improvement through diet and exercise.

When I say 'superstar body', I don't mean "here's how to look like a pro wrestler." Everybody is different, and we are all free to choose how we want to look. I chose not to be skinny anymore, to have a muscular athletic body that opened doors for my career, commanded respect and made me feel more attractive to the opposite sex (more on that later). You might not want to be as big, allowing you more mobility and endurance in your chosen sports; you may want to be bigger than I am. You may want to be ripped to shreds with tons of definition and those all-important six-pack abdominals. Or if you're female, you may want sexy and defined legs and buttocks and a slimmer waist. Whatever the case, I want you to get there. I want you to look in the mirror at your body and feel awesome. I want you to be able to dress your body up and present it in a way that makes you radiate confidence and makes people notice you.

I want you to feel like a superstar.

There will be brief moments during this book where I'll talk about my career in wrestling, my time as a Gladiator or even my early life. If so, it's for the purpose of describing how my life shaped my body and vice versa. But this is not an autobiography; it's a fitness and nutrition book. Quite frankly, who wants to hear the 'life story' of a guy who isn't even 30? The main reason I have included a few autobiographical accounts is so you, the reader, can get a glimpse of my experience in that life and understand the personality behind this book. There's also a practical reason; all too often I read fitness books and the authors omit their real life, which to me makes it hard to relate to the advice. If you're going to master your own superstar body, you have to master your personality; embrace who you are and what drives you. With that being said, I promise I won't talk about myself too much!

There will be times in the book where I talk about certain foods, supplements and products. I don't want you to feel like I'm subliminally trying to sell you anything, so I want to be 100% honest from the beginning. As of this writing, I have sponsorships with Bulletproof Nutrition and Natural Stacks. I don't receive any money from them, just a steady supply of great supplements and foods. I have also received some freebies from the generous folks at P28 Foods and Lo-Back Trax. I will give an honest recommendation where I see fit, whether it's a company I have a relationship with or not. Nobody has paid me to feature their products in the book, or even discussed the possibility with me.

I opted not to fill this book with pictures of me performing exercise demonstrations. In the modern era, almost anyone likely to read this is familiar with the vast majority of the exercises described. However, if at any time you feel like a refresher, or you are uncertain about a certain exercise, you can check out www.EXRX. net, a great site with a huge glossary of exercises and moving GIFS of almost all of them. This site, and all others described in this book can be linked to from the Superstar Body Website www.superstarbodybook. com and as always, if you are uncertain, please don't be foolish, ask for help and consult a qualified trainer.

Prologue

January 31st, 2014: The TNA Impact Wrestling event was in full flow, and after appearing in the first segment of the TV show, in a face-to-face war of words with MVP, I rushed back to the dressing room to put on my brand new gear that Jolene, the seamstress that makes all my wrestling attire, had made for me; a black with gold and silver trim version of my existing trunks and knee pad covers. I had waited until this night to debut the new attire, as this was a big night for me, and for my opponent, Chad Lail, better known as Gunner. For me, it was the first time that a British wrestler would defend a world title of a major US promotion in the UK. For Gunner, it was his first real main event with a lot of focus and time dedicated to the match and to him. He knew he had to deliver. But more importantly to both of us, it was our chance to represent the new generation of talent and the portion of young hungry guys in the dressing room who were counting on us to show that we were ready to lead a promotion.

It had been a brutal day; we were already all running on empty after a lack of sleep coming off back-to-back shows in Dublin and Glasgow, which included a 4am wake-up call to make our 6am flight. Then I had willed myself to get up early to have breakfast with my brother Ed, his wife Louisa and my two-year-old nephew Pepe. It was the only chance I was going to get to see them for probably a year.

With a ladder match earlier in the night, numerous backstage segments to shoot, and in-ring promos to think about, Gunner and I hadn't had much time to discuss anything, and by the time I was dressed for our match, we were both getting antsy; we had about 45 minutes to prepare for a match that was going to receive a lot of focus and had the potential to make or break us in a political, cut-throat industry where there is always a plethora of established guys just waiting for you to screw it up so they can move into the top spot. Every opponent I had wrestled since becoming champion had been way more established than me, so despite the ratings going up (their best in two years) the credit always naturally falls with the bigger name. This match would be the first opportunity I had to go out and tear the house down with a guy who was less established than me and make him look like a star, something I took seriously as a performer and as world champion, as I believe that is the key responsibility of being champion. I also respected Chad and wanted him to be right up there with me in the main event picture.

We discussed the match with our agent, Al Snow, and our referee, Brian Hebner. The exhaustion, nerves and frustration were taking their toll. We were fried. We were both drawing mental blanks and stumbling over our thoughts until we were both getting angry and exasperated. Al was doing his best to help us keep it together and Brian was sitting pensively, waiting for his key points. A referee is so vital in matches like this and Brian is the guy I want before anyone else. Finally I just had to mentally re-set.

"All right, Chad, let's just stop for a second. Start again, you have your big stuff, we've got the back end laid out. We've got the finish. If you trust me, let me take care of the front end of the match out there, do you trust me?"

"Of course, man," Gunner replied.

"OK, in the first half we're going to trust our instincts and go back to basics. You're awesome, I've got plenty of faith we'll nail it."

In TV wrestling, sticking to your allotted time is so important, and I was worried about meeting our time cues without missing the vital parts of the story we wanted to tell. For the first time in my career, I asked Al and Brian if we could devise a list of five or six 'key words' that would trigger Chad and I if we had another brain fart out there. We all stood together, Chad and I describing the main highlights of the match and then giving them a key word, which Al could say to Brian in his earpiece if I asked for it. It seems over-complicated but at the time it was a way to simplify communication but most importantly give me and Chad peace of mind and a confidence boost, which I'm not ashamed to admit that we needed. Al Snow, to his credit, was totally receptive to this approach and helped us as much as he could with ideas. He knew how exhausted we were and I think he could see in both of us how badly we wanted this to be good, and he wanted it to be good too.

I looked in the full length mirror and slapped on a little baby oil, re-applied my wrist tape and fixed my hair before grabbing the world title belt and marching through the halls of the Manchester Arena and into the backstage area. Visualising the match in my mind's eye, I jogged around the other wrestlers all sitting around a TV monitor watching the action in the ring. I looked at the board: one more segment and then we were up. Ten minutes to warm up and focus. A few push-ups, squats, curls and lateral raises with resistance bands and a few good isometric flexes and I was pumped up and ready to go out and look the part as world champion. As the minutes slipped away before our match, a few of the guys came over to wish us luck and give us words of encouragement. TNA president Dixie Carter and head of talent and production John Gaburick, simply known as 'Big', were at the entrance way to watch and give us some final good luck words. As the guys came through the curtain after the match before us ended, I could see Chad visualising the match one last time. This was a big night for both of us, and we didn't have it easy. I put my hand on his shoulder and said, "Let's talk out there, think slowly and tear the house down! We've got this, bud!"

Chad forced a smile through a focused expression and exploded through the curtain. Now I was 30 seconds away from my entrance. No turning back now! In an instant, images danced in my mind of me picking up my first barbell in my bedroom at 12 years old, the first protein shake I ever drank, turning down invitations to parties in high school so I could go to the gym instead, the hundreds, maybe thousands, of hours spent reading muscle magazines, books and websites. My first day of wrestling school, endless hours in a car or ring van, wrestling in a field in front of 12 people, puking at the *Gladiators* auditions, the day Dixie Carter called me and offered me a contract, my *Impact* debut, winning the world title, they had led me to this moment. The nervousness of the situation gave way to excitement and confidence; I was going to show the world that I had arrived. Almost ten years before, a nervous, lean 17-year-old kid went to his first day at wrestling school. On this night, the same nervous kid was 27, and was about to defend the Heavyweight Championship of the World. In my last seconds as 'Nick', I said one thing to myself.

"I guess I must have done something right."

I stepped through the curtain, my music blaring, lights on me and thousands of wrestling fans just like me reacting to the arrival. To be a world champion of a promotion, regardless of for how long, or under what circumstances, is an honour and a privilege. It means you're the torch bearer, the number one guy. In that moment I realised that the decisions and sacrifices I had made as a young adult had allowed me to be in that rare position.

Ever since I first picked up a barbell, I've always had a voice in the back of my mind wondering aloud if I'm doing things correctly. As I've been fortunate enough to be around so many incredible athletes and trainers over the years, I tried to soak up as much as I could, always evolving. Every day I try to ask myself, "What can I do today that helps me get to where I want to be tomorrow?"

The only answer that is applicable every day?

"Work out and eat well."

Introduction

I thought Kurt was 'ribbing' me, a term used in wrestling to mean making fun or playing a joke on someone.

I was standing near the 'go' position, the area immediately backstage behind the entrance ramp with the big screens where we make our TV entrance for *Impact*. I was getting ready for a match so I was oiled, tanned, pumped and TV-ready. I always took my presentation very seriously, it's without question one of the reasons I got an opportunity at such a young age, how I was able to work with some of the best in the world at 22 years old, and how I was able to learn from that and improve my skills. It's also one of the reasons I was considered a viable candidate for the position I was in at that time: the World Heavyweight Champion, the first Brit to ever do it.

Despite the fact that I was the champion, I was (and still am) in awe of Kurt Angle. The only Olympic gold medallist in pro wrestling became the world's best pro wrestler and will forever be indelibly etched in history as an icon of what we do. I used to study hours of Kurt Angle matches as a teenager and still to this day find it hard to process that I am a colleague of Kurt's, which made the following conversation so memorable to me.

"Mags, you're always in great shape. What do you do, man?"

I just stared at him.

"You're asking *me*? But you're Kurt Angle."

Now I should point out that I consider Kurt a friend and mentor but it still didn't make this less surreal. It was a moment I'll never forget because I was able to step outside of myself for a moment and assess where I was in life. No matter what happens in the turbulent and cruel life of a pro wrestler, one thing that is absolutely mine and mine alone is my body. I have worked hard at it and have as much passion for fitness as I do for the wrestling business – the business in which, at that particular time, I was a world champion. Here was a guy who won a gold medal in the 1996 Olympics, has made millions of dollars and inspired millions of people around the world, and he's asking me what I do to be in the shape I'm in?

I guess I'm doing something right.

Muscle has always been part of my consciousness.

I was born in 1986 in King's Lynn, an isolated port town in West Norfolk. I grew up in Docking, a small village about 15 miles outside of King's Lynn where I was the youngest of five siblings. As a small rural village in Norfolk, there wasn't much to do in Docking by way of entertainment except for playing football (soccer) on the park directly opposite our house. We would play tennis in the summer and every Friday my parents took me to the local construction college to swim at their pool, sometimes I would swim twice a week. Looking back, I realise how fortunate I was to grow up in a safe neighbourhood, with lots of space to run around and play sports and get tons of fresh air. At the time, I was always frustrated that we didn't live in a city or town, where there were more fun things to do and more people to hang out with. But I wouldn't change my upbringing one bit, especially when I consider how the environment I grew up in gave me my most valuable tool as a kid; my imagination.

From as early as I can remember, I lived vicariously through my heroes on TV: *Ghostbusters*, *Teenage Mutant Ninja Turtles* (my mother made me and my brother costumes including brown shells made from an old couch), Manchester United legend Ryan Giggs, *Gladiators* and even Eric Clapton, holding a broom handle and pretending to play guitar in jam-packed arenas watching all the VHS tapes of his concerts that my parents had. I knew what pro wrestling was and, like seemingly all kids in that era, I knew all the names of the stars, their finishing moves and their unique characteristics. The unusual thing was that we didn't have satellite television when I was growing up, so my knowledge of the product was based solely on the annuals and the toys. I would occasionally get to see clips on TV but it wasn't until my friends started recording the shows and bringing them to my house to watch in their entirety that I realised that this was more than just something I enjoyed. I was mesmerised by wrestling; the athleticism, the theatrics, the music and the muscles. Bret Hart, Sting, The British Bulldogs, Randy Savage, Hulk Hogan, Ultimate Warrior and, later, The Rock, Triple H, Steve Austin and The Undertaker all captivated my imagination and hooked me.

According to my sister, I had been talking about building my body since I was a small child, but I can only remember seriously formulating the thought after falling in love with wrestling. I've always been an independent thinker and have always been comfortable doing things on my own. At age twelve, I knew I was too young to learn to wrestle, but it wasn't going to stop me getting ready for my career. So I started doing push-ups and sit-ups in my room. We had these old weighted door stops that looked like miniature versions of the acme weights you see on Tom and Jerry cartoons, I think they were about 15lbs, so I had two of those that I would do curls, presses, lateral raises and all kinds of other stuff with. As I progressed I wanted real equipment, so I flipped through the Argos catalogue (how cool was that when you were a kid?) and instead of my previous circled items of remote controlled cars, new backpacks and footballs, I found a home barbell and dumbbell set for twenty-five pounds (about forty US dollars) and saved up my money from the after-school job I had at a fruit and vegetable store in my village.

I lied to my parents when we got to town; we had gone to King's Lynn to do some shopping, and I had told them I needed to go to Argos to get some stationery for school and would meet them back at the car. I was going to Argos, yes, but not to get school supplies. I was going to buy the barbell and dumbbell set I had been eyeing in the catalogue and saving for. I was thirteen, and like all teenage boys I thought I was James Bond when it came to lying to my parents, although in hindsight, they must have thought I was buying a lot of school supplies to come in such a big box, and for me to be struggling so much with it! I'm pretty sure they didn't believe me, but they never said anything. My dad even offered to help me carry it up to my room. That's the way they raised me and my siblings; let us make our own decisions and choose our own paths. If my parents didn't know what I had bought that day, they found out soon enough, when the incessant banging and thudding from my room upstairs became too much for my mother. She walked in to see what the hell was going on and found me with a barbell in my hands, red-faced from exertion and embarrassment (definitely more of the latter).

"Nicholas, what are you doing?" she asked.

"Um, well, I *was* doing bicep curls, but now, nothing," was my charismatic teenage response.

I became defensive, being a typical adolescent ass, because my mum was trying to dissuade me from lifting weights. I assumed she thought I was too young, or that I didn't know what I was doing, or that bodybuilding was bad for you. What I realise now that I didn't realise then was that actually she knew I was self-conscious, because the phrase she kept using was "you don't *need* to do that," not "*don't* do that." My father had a different perspective on it, being a former rugby player and a strong supporter of his children's athletic endeavours. Instead, he simply said to make sure I did it right. He would go on to give me the same advice when we talked about me becoming a pro wrestler: "Do it, but just make sure you do your best and do it right."

My mother was right, I was self-conscious.

I was skinny, puny and unimpressive. I was good at sports, but was starting to lack strength and physical presence in comparison to my older classmates (I was skipped a year of high school). This was why I was scared of people knowing I was working out, it was never my reason for working out in the first place. I don't believe that proving people wrong should ever be your main reason for doing something, even though I have been guilty of it myself. I was captivated by pro wrestling, and the idea of being a pro wrestler, and that meant looking like my heroes. I didn't want to be skinny any more, and I knew in my heart from day one that I was going to change that. I vividly remember after about three months of training, getting changed in the dressing room of the sports hall for PE, and one of my friends saying, "Whoa, Nick's got pecs!" (My chest was the first muscle to really respond well to my training.) I felt immediately vindicated, knowing that I was right, and more importantly I felt confident and excited, because I knew this was only the beginning...

We all have our passions in life; most become hobbies, something you watch or follow, or something you pursue. If you're lucky, you can make your passion your livelihood; your career. I have felt that lucky for the last ten years, while I have earned my living thanks to professional wrestling. Although I still have a lot of goals within my business that I want to achieve, I can (and do) take pride in the fact that I have reached some already. I feel the same way about writing this book. I recently realised that for as long as I have dreamed about being a sports entertainer, I have also dreamed about having a better physique, trying to look like all those guys you see in the magazines or in the movies or, in my case, at arenas in front of thousands and on television captivating the imaginations of millions around the world. At first, bodybuilding was just a necessary endeavour: to look the part in order to be a wrestler. But immediately it became a passion in its own right, something that just happened to be necessary to my career. I guess I'm doubly lucky in that respect; I get to dedicate my life to my passion, something I urge you all to do as well. I was passionate enough to pursue a qualification in the field as a Certified Personal Trainer, while enjoying my career as a pro wrestler. When I had a chance to reflect on it, I realised that I had in fact achieved goals with my body and my career without even noticing; not only am I a sports entertainer, but I've appeared in fitness magazines, I've acted, I write for a magazine, I've appeared on television in front of millions...and I feel like I've barely scratched the surface.

I decided to write this book after receiving a lot of emails, letters, tweets and Facebook messages from people asking how to improve their bodies. It took me a long time to realise, but thanks to all the people who have reached out to me, and the people close to me making me aware of it, I understand now that maybe I do have some good advice to offer. I don't claim to be an expert, or full of wisdom, but I can tell you what works for me, what I know works for others, and my understanding of why.

And I intend to show it to you in simple, no-nonsense sections. This book will not be full of unnecessary information or gimmicks, but it also won't insult your intelligence, and will hopefully give you what you need to know in order to help you in your own pursuit of a better body.

I believe there are few greater feelings in the world than improving your body; the first time you look in the mirror and notice abs, the first time you realise how much easier that last run was, the first time somebody notices how your sleeves are now tighter, these feelings will empower you and reward you for all your hard work. And, if you're anything like me, will spur you on to achieve even greater gains.

What to expect in this book

As I alluded to earlier, I don't claim to be all-knowing when it comes to fitness and nutrition. In my opinion, nobody is. That's why I enlisted the opinions and expertise of the incredible men and women who have contributed to this book, because I am not arrogant enough to think that my advice is the only advice you will need or want. What I'm going to give you in this book is the best advice I can give, based on what I have seen work for me and others, for gaining muscle mass, burning body fat and improving your performance and your wellbeing.

I'll give you facts from results, not research: when I read some fitness books, magazines or blogs, I am stunned at the amount of advice that is given based on an irrelevant study at a university somewhere that somebody then interprets to create some fad diet, fad exercise plan or, worse, both. These things will inevitably go around in circles, contradicting themselves and repeating themselves; 'stop stretching' will be followed by 'do more stretching', 'eggs will kill you' followed by 'the egg diet', 'low-fat beach body diet' followed by 'eat fat, get thin'... Enough already! Don't get me wrong, I find this kind of thing interesting as some casual coffee table reading, it just doesn't give you the fundamental knowledge of how to have a better body. I will do my best to do that in this book.

If you take nothing else away from this book, please take this: knowledge is power, and that phrase has never been truer than here.

That's why I ask you to read this book from cover to cover at least once, then refer to sections as and when you need them. I've tried to make this a reference book as much as possible, so when you need a refresher or just some inspiration, you can grab it and look at it quickly and get on with your life. But at least once, read the whole thing. You'll be glad you did if you are serious about getting the body you want. When *you* know the key fundamental principles of working out and eating right, *you and you alone are now in control*, the power to change is in your hands. I want to show you how to integrate working out and eating for a better body into your real life, and show you that it won't be as huge a culture shock as you might think. I want you to work for the body that you are proud of. I want to put the power in your hands.

I want to emphasise my mantra in this book:

TRAIN

EAT

LIVE

When I say this, it's because so many people I have seen place too much emphasis and pressure on their body from purely the aesthetic point of view. There are a lot of people in the world who look great on the outside but are a disaster on the inside. Believe me, you can tell the difference; it's in our DNA to instinctively identify people who are vibrant, healthy and fit. That comes from more than just big muscles or low body fat. It comes from radiating a sense of health and wellbeing that will ultimately allow you to look your best for life, not just for short periods of time. Sometimes people will see me and they will ask "How do you train?", "What do you eat?" – sometimes even "What are you taking?" (!)

What I wish they would ask is "How do you live?"

Let's get started.

10 To Remember

I'm not a big believer in information overload; we only get one life, I don't believe in spending too much of it processing unnecessary information, especially when the information is to help me reach a goal. Just give me the essential information or tools; if I choose to delve deeper I will. I encourage you to do the same, not only in your information accrual for improving your body, but in your methods.

Health and fitness is a multi-billion dollar industry, which is both good and bad: good because it means there are more gyms than ever, more supplement stores than ever, more magazines and books than ever and it's never been easier to eat right while travelling; bad because in addition to all the good things available, there are even more useless and time-wasting things out there, especially in the publications area. You can get so overwhelmed with useless information that you can't hold on to the important stuff, or worse still, you don't even know it because the magazines and websites don't want you to know the most important stuff, because then you might not buy any more of their products. I'm going to try and give you the need-to-know items that I believe to be the most essential in every area. Before I do that, I'm going to give you what I call the '10 To Remember'. Why? Because I want you to have the necessary information and be able to identify the unnecessary information, and throw this crap away before you try and take on new information. Plus, everybody loves a good top ten.

1. **Don't ignore the fundamentals.**

   Every time I go to the gym, I see somebody peering at an open magazine or a printed page on the floor then haphazardly attempting a one-legged squat balancing on a BOSU ball with a kettle bell raise and I wonder when the last time was that they actually did a real squat. These magazines and personal trainers feed people's desires to have everything as fast as possible by suggesting these moves that 'combine two exercises in one', when in reality it's more like doing half of each. Of all the people that ask me for advice, I'd say at least two-thirds of them could gain 5lbs of muscle and probably lose a couple of per cent body fat just from doing squats, deadlifts, bench press and pull-ups for a month. The same holds true with diet. I'll see guys taking all kinds of supplements, or making special recipes, or eating nothing but rice for a day or whatever it might be, then when I ask them about if they know about macros, or calorie cycling, or even a good ratio of protein/carbs/fats, they look at me like I asked them to recite the Magna Carta. Understand the fundamentals, then choose what else you want to try to digest. To use a car analogy, don't try and put Ferrari wheels on a Ford Escort chassis. Develop a great base with solid fundamentals, then you have the power to change your body to fit whatever look you want.

2. **"I don't want to get too big."**

   Shut up. This is one of the most irritating things I hear when people ask me for advice. They'll point to a magazine with an IFBB pro on the cover and say, "I want to add some muscle but I don't want to look like that," to which I reply, "Don't worry, you couldn't even if you wanted to." Then I usually end my conversation with that person. Remember this; everything that is being pushed in fashionable magazines and websites today was common knowledge in bodybuilding about twenty years earlier. Respect bodybuilding, even if you don't follow the culture. I don't care for the culture of powerlifting, but I follow the advice for increasing strength and I respect the experts in the field. Apply the same open-mindedness to every genre and you will open so many possibilities to improve yourself.

3. **Think like a sculptor.**
    Points one and two both tie in with this. The following sentence may be the most valuable sentence in the book: *the key to improving your physique is to add quality mass in the form of lean muscle, then chisel down until you reach your desired look.* So many people flip-flop between trying to add muscle then getting frustrated at looking soft and trying to burn fat. I have friends who are skinny-fat, then they decide they want abs for the summer and do tons of crunches, planks, Swiss ball pull-ins and whatever else is in their 'six weeks to beach-ready abs' article and I'll say, "You realise that in order to have visible abdominals you'll have to lose about fifteen pounds?" And they look at me like I just asked them for one of their kidneys. If you're stuck in a rut or you've reached a plateau, just keep going back to that premise, think like a sculptor. Add the mass, then chisel it down.

4. **Diet/Exercise, 50/50.**
    All too often, improvements are slowed by a lop-sided dedication to diet or exercise. In my experience, people trying to lose weight typically tend to focus too hard on diet and don't work out effectively, while people trying to add muscle get lazy with their diet and, as Steve Austin has said on his 'Unleashed' podcast, "You can't out-train a shitty diet!" Obviously these are

typical examples but the point is that your body's physical and hormonal response to food and exercise is the same, but both are enhanced by the other. You can tip the scales one way or another, just make sure you return the balance. If you have a bad diet day you can increase your cardio that day, or if you didn't bring your A-game in the gym that day, make sure you eat clean that day and eat the right stuff to trigger a hormonal response. But strive to maintain a 50/50 balance between the construction (exercise) and raw materials (diet).

5. **By failing to prepare, you are preparing to fail.**
Benjamin Franklin isn't somebody you usually quote when you're talking about having six-pack abs and mountainous biceps, but this iconic quote rings very true when it comes to your physique. When it comes to diet, preparation is easily one of the most important ingredients for success. My rice cooker is one of my most prized possessions; I cook up a big batch and cook up a batch of lean meat like turkey patties, ground beef, chicken breasts or whatever I have, and usually some kind of veggies like roast vegetables, box up individual portions in food containers and I have a load of physique-fuelling meals ready to go. When it comes to training, prepare yourself to get the most out of that valuable time in the gym. Plan your workout, include a plan B in case of unavailable equipment, take your supplements in adequate time to digest them, have your post-workout fuel ready and be mentally prepared to get the work done. Both Arnold Schwarzenegger and Frank Zane, two of my favourite physiques of all time, have professed the importance of preparation and visualisation before a workout.

Superstar Spotlight – Mickie James

First off I would like to say thank you to Nick for asking me to be a part of his book. I think we all will benefit from the vast amount of fitness knowledge he has provided here. His passion, dedication, and love for the world of all fitness is truly a motivator for me, as I hope it is for all of you.

I think one of the hardest things for me was to get back in shape after having my son, Donovan. There are days I still struggle with this. As we all know babies can be very demanding. I went from working out for two hours almost every day, to now one hour of actual gym time about three, sometimes four days a week if I'm lucky. So this is for all the mommas and papas out there – "Maximise Your Minutes!"

Before you even walk into that gym set your mind on a purpose. Clear your mind of everything except your body. Walk in with a mission – a mission to kill it! If you can do that I promise you that you will achieve in one hour what so many take three hours to even remotely compare.

I think for many people they think, "Well, I'm at the gym so that's a step in the right direction." And it is, so I commend you for that. But walking on the treadmill while texting and playing on Facebook is not effective cardio. And working out in a group of five with five-minute breaks in between your sets, chit-chatting the entire time you're in the gym is not what I call working out. It actually is working against yourself because you allow time for your body to cool down too much, which makes you prone to more injuries, and you will hardly see any significant changes.

When I go to the gym it's all business...I'm not there to socialise. Fact I'm probably the most unapproachable when I'm at the gym with my head down and geared up ready to go. And that's not because I'm trying to be an asshole, but because I'm there to work, because being healthy is part of my job, a job that I take very seriously.

First take a deep breath, focus, and get ready to kick it in! Your mindset will dictate your whole workout. Start off from a great place and finish in a better one!

I always warm up with 15min of good cardio to get the blood flowing and body moving. Then I finish with 20-30min of strong cardio. I'm not talking about just getting on the machine and hitting QuickStart. I mean really push yourself. Get the energy up and set the pace for the rest of your workout. Change intensity, resistance, and speed to really kick it up. Don't be afraid to push your limits and break a sweat! And this particularly is more for the workout part – don't worry what everyone else is thinking about you! You are there for you – no-one else but YOU!

I've included a few sample routines of different workouts that work for me. As you will notice I am the queen of supersets! For me it keeps me moving so

I'm burning fat while I'm building muscle. Plus the fact I'm usually on a bit of a cramped schedule at the moment means it's the best way for me to make sure I get a solid workout in and maximise every minute I get in there.

LEGS
1) Leg extensions superset with Hamstring curls ~ 10 360 jump squats
   (3 sets of 12-15 4th set drop set 10 each)
2) smith machine ~ squats and Hindu squats supersets 3 of 15 each ~ calf raises 3 sets of 20
3) lunges 3 sets of 15-20
   2 min jump rope in between
4) dead lifts 3 sets of 12-15 into 10 box jumps

GLUTES
1) I do the same superset as I do to start my leg routine. Instead of the 360 jumps I'll switch to kettle bell cross overs
2) The butt blaster or banded kick backs 3 sets of 15-20 ~ 20 kettle bell squats
3) single leg balance with kettle bell 3 sets of 10 each leg
4) in and outer thigh machine [I prefer the ankle wrap on the universal machine] 3 sets of 20 ~ 20 side to side jumping lunges

BACK and BI's
1) superset lat pull downs 4 sets of 15 change hands position each set into biceps 21's
2) superset free weight single arm row into double back flyes ~ 3 sets or 15 each

3) Superset Bent over rows ~ switch grip into bicep curls ~ 3 sets of 15 each
4) standing lunge universal machine row with the double rope into knee lifts 3 sets of 15
5) superset Bent over back flyes into Arnold single arm curls 3 sets of 15

CHEST and TRI's
1) Chest press 3 sets of 15. 4th drop set ~ 20 burpees in between each
2) Superset push-ups (change push-up for more of a challenge) into tricep pushdowns. 3 sets of 15
3) triple set with bar chest press into skull crusher into laying pull overs. At least 10-20reps each exercise straight into the next.
4) Superset free weight chest flyes into tricep extinctions
5) 4 sets of Dips into 1min mountain climbers

SHOULDERS and CORE
1) 4 sets of 20 lateral raises
2) shoulder press 3 sets of 15
3) Superset shoulder raises into kettle bell side twists 3 sets of 15
4) Shrugs into side bends 3 sets of 15
5) Plank/ side plank *hold each as long as you can

Also I swear by yoga. If I could do it every day I would. I know some people that it's their only form of exercise and they are in incredible shape. Yoga challenges you and your muscles to think and react differently than any other exercise out there. It also is a key element for me to keep my body in alignment as well as my head. I recommend it to anyone and *everyone. You should try to incorporate it into your weekly workout regime at least once a week.*

I also tend to work out abs every other day about 5-10 min at the end of my workout. It's usually about 2-3 exercises or 50-100 reps. Then with whatever time I have left I blast intense cardio.

I try to do something physical every day. Whether you make it to the gym or not it's best for your mind, body, and spirit to get outside and get your body moving. Join a class, take the dog for a jog, go ride your bike, anything! You will just feel so much better about you.

Mickie James is one of the most decorated Female Professional Wrestlers of all time. Former WWE Divas Champion, 5-time WWE Women's Champion and 3-time TNA Knockouts Champion. She is also a recording artist, her latest album 'Somebody's Gonna Pay' is available on iTunes.
Twitter: @MickieJames
Facebook: facebook.com/MickieLJames
Instagram: @themickiejames
Website: www.MickieJames.com

6. **Get in. Get it done. Get out.**

The effectiveness of your workout is not determined by how much time you spend in the gym, but by how much stimulation you subjected your body to while you were training. A lot of people fall into the habit of giving themselves a set amount of time to work out and conclude that results will come based on that time dedication. Not true. In fact, spending too long in the gym can be just as detrimental to your physique aspirations as not spending enough time. I don't care if you're a gym rat, an aspiring pro athlete, a mechanic or a stay-at-home parent, **take it seriously.** Maximise your minutes in the gym or wherever you train. Push yourself to achieve the effective amount of stimulation required to trigger a response from your body.

Some of my best workouts have come from having limited time, and blasting a body part with limited rest periods in between sets. This is where preparation is key; planning how I can do the effective amount to trigger a response in say, 40 minutes for a back workout. Do what you need to do in order to trigger a response from your body, anything you do after that is not helping. Get in. Get it done. Get out.

7. Don't be embarrassed.

I worked out with a cheap in-home barbell and dumb-bell set in my bedroom for the first year because I was too embarrassed of my physique (or lack thereof) to go to a gym. But after I dedicated myself to it and started to see improvements, I finally got the courage to go to a local gym. I was always self-conscious of my body, but more importantly, of looking like I didn't know what I was doing. Knowing what I know now, I realise how silly that was, and what a waste of focus. Years, and thousands of hours in gyms later, I realise that I'm now the guy that 14-year-old me was afraid of looking foolish in front of.

But guess what? I don't see you in the gym, I don't see anyone, because I'm too concerned with my own work-out. Don't let fear of looking like a novice stop you from hitting the gym, trying new things and pushing yourself. We were all there once. Nobody is looking at you.

8. **Worship the mirror, not the scales.**

We are all born with different bone structures, different muscle bellies, different adipose tissue, different hormonal responses, different everything. It's one of the fascinating and brilliant things about life and about the human body. So if there are over six billion different bodies on planet earth, that makes you one in over six billion.

One in six billion.

So why would you ever let somebody tell you what your ideal weight is? BMI (Body Mass Index) is complete and utter nonsense. According to the BMI, at six feet four inches tall and averaging around 250lbs, I am obese. I'm not obese. I know guys who weigh the same as I do and are 5'10". And they're not obese. They have muscle mass and greater bone density, but they're not obese. Unless your career requires you to be a specific weight, or you have been advised by a doctor to lose weight to aid your joints, forget how much you weigh. It doesn't matter. What matters is how you feel, and in the context of this book, how you look. I have never heard a guy notice a hot girl and say "wow, look at her, she must only weigh 110lbs!" Similarly, I've never heard a girl say "I used to think Dwayne 'The Rock' Johnson was hot until I found out he's obese." Check yourself out in the mirror; it's not vanity, it's close monitoring of your progress. I don't own a set of scales, and never have.

9. **Set goals.**

While your mind can always be tuned in to the top of the mountain, your brain needs to be planning realistic stages to reach in order to reach your ultimate goal. Set yourself monthly, weekly, even daily goals. Each time you conquer a task you set for yourself, I promise your motivation will increase. This is especially true when you're a beginner. I loved being new to weight training and nutrition, you make such incredible gains, it feels fantastic. Trust me, the better you get, the harder it is to make improvements, and that's when the real work begins. Guess what? There is no mountain top. Self-improvement is an endless pursuit, so keep setting goals and you will become the image you dream of for yourself.

10. If you're not evolving, you're revolving.

"Learning never exhausts the mind." – *Leonardo Da Vinci* I'm very fortunate to have met and worked with some incredible people who are much more qualified than me. Whether it be Olympic athletes, IFBB champion body-builders, CEOs of multi-million dollar companies, nutrition gurus or best-selling authors, I have access to great information that I can apply to my own life and attempt to improve myself. As I alluded to in the previous point, the quest for a better body never ends, which means that every day there are new studies, new techniques being pioneered, new breakthroughs in nutrition that smash the old beliefs. This is where the online and magazine reading is a useful tool for your success. It's vital to have an understanding of the base knowledge first, but then you have all these avenues open to you to explore; enhancing performance, increasing focus, improving sleep, achieving a better sex life and the best part is, it changes all the time. *You have to keep your body guessing.* Once your body starts to get used to stimuli, it no longer needs to improve to adapt. Survival of the fittest requires one to evolve, to keep up. Every time your phone, tablet, or computer tells you to update, you do it. Your body is the most complex piece of equipment you will ever own. Update it.

Part 1

TRAIN

On the mountains of truth you can never climb in vain: either you will reach a point higher up today, or you will be training your powers so that you will be able to climb higher tomorrow – Friedrich Nietzsche

I debated on which order I should write the main body of this book. As you can see, I've divided the book into three sections, the mantra I try to live by: *Train. Eat. Live.* I could have placed the sections in any order and the information could still be relevant. But let's cut the crap: When I read a fitness book, as much as I agree that diet, exercise and lifestyle are equally important, I go straight to the workouts. So I figured I'll put TRAIN at the beginning.

To me, there are few greater feelings in the world than the feeling you get after you know you've completed a really good training session. There's scientific relevance to this; your body releases endorphins, which are neurotransmitters released by the brain and act as your body's natural stress and pain relief. Think about that; when you work out, your body instantly rewards you with feel-good chemicals that you won't get arrested for. Everything happens for a reason; that's your body telling you, "More of this, please."

The reason that the TRAIN section of this book is arguably the most important is economics. Let's say you dedicate 90 minutes of your day to your workout, then you have to maximise those minutes to get the results you want. If you waste them, you have to wait until the next day for another bite of the apple. Diet and lifestyle are ongoing and fall into the other 22.5 hours of your day. You have to make your workout count.

Where?

Choosing your workspace and making the most of it are two different things. First of all, I appreciate that not all of you reading this will get the luxury of being able to 'choose' where you work out. There may only be one gym in your town, college, school, office, apartment complex etc, in which case, you may have to supplement with at-home training. But if you are fortunate enough to have a choice, these are my key elements to look for when choosing a regular gym:

- Good selection of free weights: While there are some incredible machines out there, ultimately I know if they have a good range of barbells, dumbbells and Olympic bars, I can get a great workout.

- Space to play with: To really get the most out of your body you need to set it free with movements that require some space. Olympic lifts, farmer's walk, box jumps and kettle bell swings aren't fun when you're constantly having to mind your surroundings. Many gyms now have a designated open area with equipment in the corners that can be brought into the middle and returned when not in use.

- Climate control: This may seem neurotic, but some gyms get their working temperature very wrong. One of my favourite gyms, Gold's Gym in St Petersburg, Florida, has great air conditioning, but as the temperature outside dropped off, they would open their big shutter doors and let fresh air in, maintaining a healthy sweat temperature of around 70-73 degrees. Some gyms (especially in the summer) go way overboard with their air conditioning making it difficult to get some heat and pliability in your muscles and you can't get a healthy sweat going. On the other end of the spectrum, stifling humidity is also uncomfortable and hinders your training.

- Mirrors: You have to get the idea out of your head that checking yourself out in the mirror in the gym is vain. You have to be able to monitor your progress so you know what is working and what is not. Also, there is no better time to see your gains than when you have a pump (when blood has rushed to your muscle bellies and the muscle is swollen as a result). On top of that, you need to be able to check your form at all times. This is especially true with free weight exercises: making sure you are balanced, strict and engaging the right muscle groups.

- Atmosphere: What kind of atmosphere you want to train in is completely your call. Some people want the shiny, attractive health club with all the creature comforts, rows of gleaming machines, dressing rooms that look like a cigar bar and pretty people that seem to materialise on cue. Others want the spit'n'sawdust gym with cast iron plates that are older than most of the people lifting them, chalk dust adorning most of the floor and a continuous soundtrack of clanging weights, screams of exertion and music proclaiming some kind of pain or hate. My personal preference is somewhere in the middle. I need there to be a serious nature to the gym; a desire to push yourself and take training seriously. But I also want the facilities to be clean and inviting. If I feel good, I train hard. I don't want to waste my energy with worrying about upsetting the clientele with my training methods, nor do I want to be judged by a bunch of power lifters for training my 'mirror muscles'. In my experience, Gold's Gyms tend to get the balance right almost everywhere in the world. But there are thousands of fantastic independent gyms all over the world as well as smaller, high-performance training centres with great trainers that are really gaining popularity. The key is to find a gym with an atmosphere that makes you want to better yourself; there is no wrong answer.

When?

The question of when to train is one of the most frequently asked. It makes sense to want to know this; after all, as I alluded to earlier, you need to maximise your time in the gym so it's natural to want to know when the body is most primed to do so.

Arnold Schwarzenegger (my biggest inspiration in fitness and nutrition) professed his preference to train in the morning, particularly as he got older, so that the rest of his day was free to tackle the mountain of tasks that a life like his consists of. Back in his heyday, Arnold would often train twice per day, something I have been known to do myself from time to time, but I don't recommend it for beginners. Arnold trained that way when he was a full-time pro, so he spent the rest of his day eating, recuperating and preparing. Similarly, I have the advantage of being paid to be an athlete, so if I'm not wrestling or travelling, I will often train abs and cardio, higher rep weight training or some plyometrics in the morning, then hit the iron in the late afternoon or early evening. I always found that I have more strength and respond more positively to afternoon or evening training. I usually want to tackle my business tasks, emails, writing, bills etc early in the morning when I am alert and my brain is functioning. By the time I get to the gym, I want to be 100% focused on that and nothing else. It's another case of personal preference. Try out different times and listen to your body, see what works for you and remember that it's never set in stone; sometimes I will force myself to lift early for a couple of weeks just to keep my body guessing and see what changes it brings. Different body processes peak at different times, so keep this in mind when figuring out what works best for you:

Morning: Testosterone peaks (males). Mental alertness, memory and cognitive function peak (late morning), body temperature is low.

Afternoon: Pain tolerance peaks, adrenalin and body temperature rises, mental and physical function balances. Many people suffer a low energy point at or around noon.

Evening: Strength, stamina, coordination, lung performance, flexibility and body temperature all peak. Mental alertness can often be waning.

Night: Melatonin (sleep inducing hormone) production increases and body processes slow in preparation for sleep.

Superstar Spotlight – Nick Ehrlich

Motivation and Goal Setting

Congratulations! You are about to embark on an exciting and rewarding fitness journey that will surely show you a level of success that you have only dreamed of! Enclosed in the chapters of this book are plenty of workouts, nutrition tidbits, and guidance that will lay out a yellow-brick-road to take you from zero to hero and guide you along the smooth and steady road to your goals.

Of course, it never really works out that way, does it? How many times before have you picked up a programme just like this one, started out fast and furious, and wound up right where you started; dejected, depressed, and no leaner that you were in the first place? We have ALL experienced that feeling of falling short of a fitness or weight-loss goal, and *we all know how crushing that feeling can be when confronted with it.*

So how does one get on a plan and stick to it? How is it possible that this time will be the time that works, and that this will be when you finally give up your excuses and embrace the makings of a new, fitter, leaner you?

My website and programme Lean Life Revolution, much like Nick and his book that you're holding, is all about setting goals, refocusing energies, and achieving things previously seen as insurmountable. When talking to clients and readers, we at LLR embrace three truths involved in any goal- or challenge-based fitness routine;

The First Rule – Take Everything You "Know" And Throw It Away

If I had a dollar for every time someone told me that they "know" they can't lose weight, or they "know" they will always hate vegetables, or that they "know" that they will never be a morning person, I would be sitting on an island somewhere having my feet rubbed by my personal team of massage therapists. Starting a new lifestyle while holding on to the things that kept you from what you wanted initially is just like buying a new car and then hitting it with a baseball bat to match the dents of your old one. Now obviously you know your body, and know what your routine has been up to this point, but it's important to understand that what you "know" has got you to a place where you are physically unhappy and out of shape.

The other problem with "knowing" things is that once you open your mouth to show your knowledge, you tend to close your ears to the teachings of others. Think about it: you bought this book for a reason, to learn about new ways of training, eating, and thinking, so why would you now close yourself off to all of that expert advice because you "know" that you like doing something different? You may as well have taken the money you used to buy this book, gone to the local arcade, and played 30 games of ski-ball instead.

Think about this: when elephants are brought to the circus as babies, their legs are tied to a tent-stake that is driven into the ground a few yards away. The baby elephant is too weak to pull the stake from the earth, and eventually learns that he can't pull himself free, so it's pointless for it to try any more. As the elephant grows, the tent stake is never changed, and even after the elephant has achieved its massive size and incredible strength, it never pulls at the tent stake that it now could easily yank from the ground. This is an example of learned helplessness, a theory that explains how people or animals will eventually give up trying something if they learn enough times that they can't do it. The elephant remembers how it struggled to free itself previously, so it doesn't even attempt to pull its captor stake out of the ground in spite of the fact that it could do so with the ease that you and I could pull a petal off a flower.

Our own behaviours and knowledge can be just like that tent stake. If you have tried and failed to lose weight or get in shape previously, you may now think

that it's impossible. You may have developed some
theory about how you are supposed to be overweight,
or that you can't maintain a healthy diet, or that
you can never enjoy yourself at the gym, and much
like the elephant tied to the stake, you refuse to yank
at the rope tying you to a body and a life that are
making you unhappy.

Stop holding on to the things you "know," and start
to embrace new challenges, new ways of thinking,
and new patterns of behaviour. Once you truly
embrace these things and stop telling people what
you "know," you will be ready to achieve a whole
new level of success and growth.

The Second Rule – Embrace New Ideas and Practices
Ok, hard truth here; the way you've done thing up to
this point hasn't worked. If you had the answer, or
were engaging in best practices, then you wouldn't
have bought this book in the first place. You are here
looking for a better way of doing things, and if you're
open to them, you'll find them in the pages of this
very book.

Now I'll be the first person to say that new things
and practices are intimidating. There's no way
around it really, we as human beings are creatures
of habit, and we avoid discomfort or dissonance
at every turn, even if it means holding on to a
behaviour or activity that we know is detrimental or
dangerous. If you think about it, there are probably
several things that you are avoiding or prolonging
right now just to avoid a new or unknown behaviour
(I personally have a crippling fear of the dentist,

and routinely go way longer than I should without going, just to avoid the fear of sitting in that chair). I once heard a great joke about habits, in that they are similar to being shot in the stomach. Once the bullet is in there, the longer you wait to pull it out, the more damage it's going to cause when you do so. The longer you wait to change your behaviours, the harder it will be to do, and the more urgent changes then become.

Sure, it's uncomfortable to change things you've been doing for years, but it's only through change and struggle that we truly grow. Someone once told me, "I never learned anything about myself when stuff wasn't changing." That simple quote has guided and pushed me to constantly challenge and analyse the practices and habits in my life to make sure that everything I do has a positive effect on my total wellbeing. Much like a muscle that has been trained with resistance, we as people only grow and develop when faced with change, struggle, or resistance. The easy roads are never the ones that take us where we want to go, it's the paths that challenge and test us that lead to true success.

Try making a list of the things that you know are preventing you from being in the shape you want to be in. This can be about the things you eat, the ways you avoid exercise, ways you relax or recreate, or anything that you see as being an obstacle between you and the body of your dreams. Don't worry if the list is long either, because you are going to take it down in little pieces. Once your list is complete (for now) start with the little things that are easy fixes, such as not using creamer in your coffee or walking places in lieu of riding the bus or driving. Make these small changes one at a time, giving each one a few days to sink in before adding another. Once you have a few small changes hammered in, then start to modify the big changes that you need to make. Getting some momentum with the small fixes will help to motivate and drive you when the big fixes come up.

The Third Rule – The Journey Is The Destination

When I was a kid, I LOVED kung-fu and karate movies. I would often spend my weekends and evenings sitting on the couch watching some movie about an impetuous young man who needed to learn kung-fu or some other martial art of fighting discipline in order to defend himself from a group of bullies at his school/park/village. This young man would always find an unlikely teacher who lived somewhere in solitary isolation to teach him the secrets of martial arts, and after working with the teacher for weeks (delivered in a sweet training montage), the main character would eventually beat the snot out of his aggressor and end the movie with the girl in his arms and his fist in the air in triumph. I wish life actually worked out this way too, because any time I stood up to a bully as a kid it usually ended with me getting my ass kicked by a second bully while the first one recovered and then jumped in.

What started to fascinate me as I got older was not the young hero who won the big fight at the end of the movie, but the teachers that the main characters *would always seek out. These masters of the art would always be somewhere off by themselves where they could train, meditate, and reflect without any distractions. They never sought confrontation, or picked fights with neighbourhood bullies; they just practised, studied, and kept to themselves until the wimpy high school kid limped into their living room with a bloody nose and a need to learn karate.*

It is only now in my adult life that I realise that these masters were the real heroes of these films, as the goal for them was not to learn enough to kick someone else's ass, but to enjoy the constant and ongoing journey of knowledge, self-development, and practice. Think of Mr Miyagi in The Karate Kid *doing crane kicks at the beach: he wasn't doing them to try to blast some other guy in his apartment building in the face for stealing his newspaper every Sunday, he did it because the constant repetition and practice was meditative and rewarding for him.*

When embarking on a new training programme, and with respect to the aforementioned karate movie format, your focus should be on becoming the master and not the hero. Your goal when you go to the gym every day should not be on achieving the arms and abs of your dreams and then "being finished"; it should be on the constant and perpetual journey of getting stronger, faster, leaner, and more well-rounded as an athlete and exerciser. Your focus should always be on progress, not perfection, and the constant drive to just "get better." Every day provides a new opportunity to improve, and there are so many ways you can do so. Take some time to work on strength, then switch to flexibility, then conditioning, and so on. Constantly look for your weak points and fix them, then move on to the next weak link in your physical chain. This can seem like an insurmountable task for some, but the truly successful people in sports, fitness, or any physical endeavour are the ones who constantly locate, establish, and then work to correct their weak points. Make your fitness journey about enjoying the ride, and not just getting to a destination.

Nick Ehrlich is a trainer and coach at SWEAT Performance in Baltimore, Maryland. Nick works with everybody from part-timers to professional athletes, the walls of the gym adorned with signed thank you pictures from players in the NFL, NBA and NCAA. Nick is also the creator of Lean Life Revolution, a website and programme series dedicated to streamlining the flow of necessary information helping people achieve a sustainable lean and cut physique as quickly and smartly as possible.
Web: LeanLifeRevolution.com
Twitter: @FitnessWithNick
Instagram:@leanliferevolution
Facebook: facebook.com/leanliferevolution

Understand your Body Type

Before you start to perfect the bodywork, you have to identify the chassis that your genetics gave you. Your somatotype, more commonly referred to as your body type, is this chassis.

I don't want you to use your body type as some kind of crutch or excuse for not reaching your full potential; it drives me crazy when guys see the gains you've made from hard work, trial and error and education and then say, "I wish I had your genetics." The reason you need to identify your body type is so you know what techniques and practices to implement to best reach your desired superstar look.

Ectomorph

The Ectomorph is characterised by narrow shoulders and waist, long arms and legs, and slim muscles that taper to small joints.

If you fall more on the ectomorph portion of the scale, mass is not going to come easily; you'll have to take in a high amount of calories and generally stimulate all muscle bellies with high volume, heavy compound moves and single joint isolation exercises. The good news is that body fat is scarce on an ectomorph frame, so once you've earned some muscle mass, you'll be able to develop definition and make it visible. Plus, you may not have to be as strict with your diet when it comes to carbohydrates and fats.

Mesomorph

The Mesomorph is the perfect structure for muscle and definition; long torso, wide shoulders, slim waist and strong joints with large muscle bellies.

If you're predominantly a mesomorph, you will respond well to traditional training and diet techniques. Maintaining moderation when it comes to carbs and fats should allow you to stay lean while acquiring muscle mass. You can't be completely careless with diet; even with an ideal frame, you still need to put the work in to see the results you want. [1]

Endomorph

The Endomorph is characterised by wider waist and torso, short limbs and big joints.

---

[1] Huge thanks to Sam Shaw for this awesome artwork. Follow him at @TheSamuelShaw on Twitter and to contact him for your own custom artwork email shawdawgarts@gmail.com

The main concern if you're more endomorphic is staying lean; you're going to have to be strict with diet and cardio to stave off unwanted body fat. Strength should not be a concern, so muscle mass should come with adequate work in the weight room. The real work is going to be in chiselling down the mass when the time comes.

The important thing to remember when it comes to body types is that everybody falls somewhere between two. For example, with long limbs, small joints but decent shoulder width, I am an Ecto-Mesomorph (predominantly Ectomorph but with Mesomorphic qualities too). Analyse your body and figure out where you fall on the scale.

Make the Most of your Workout

I must govern the clock, not be governed by it – Golda Meir

Don't go into the gym with the intention of just going through the motions. An average approach to your workout will lead to an average body. Want to be average? Didn't think so. Take the time to read about these approaches and principles that will help you squeeze every drop out of the time you spend in the gym improving your body.

Superstar Spotlight – Kurt Angle

A lot of the guys remark to me about how I get so focused, and Nick for one is always complimenting me on how I can seemingly switch in an instant when it's Go-Time. While I believe that some of that ability is a blessing, I also want to point out that under the surface I am focusing constantly. All day long, I'm always thinking about what I can do to push myself to the limit. I'm always using visualisation; I think it helps me more than anything. If I have a match, I'm visualising in the car on the way to the arena. Before I train, I'm visualising what I want to achieve as I walk in to the gym. I developed my visualisation before the Olympics, where I even went as far to see a psychiatrist and hypnotherapist to put me under and do visualisation techniques; I would visualise taking my opponent down again and again to the point where I could not see any other option but victory. Over time I developed the ability to do this myself without help. So I encourage you to spend any amount of time you can spare to visualise yourself achieving your goal, whatever it may be, over and over again. Eventually, you will see no other option but your own personal victory.

Kurt Angle is one of the most decorated wrestlers in history, both amateur and professional.

As an amateur, he's a 2-time NCAA Division 1 Champion and, of course, a 1996 Olympic Gold Medallist.

As a pro, he's held just about every significant title there is to hold: WWE European Champion, Intercontinental Champion, Tag Team Champion, King of the Ring, World Heavyweight Champion, WWE Champion. IWGP Heavyweight Champion, TNA X Division Champion, Tag Team Champion, World Heavyweight Champion. His success transitioned into movies including his most notable appearance in the critically acclaimed Warrior with Tom Hardy. He also happens to be one of my heroes, so I'm blown away that he contributed to this book for me.
Website: www.KurtAngleBrand.com
Twitter: @RealKurtAngle

Mind and Muscle

The tryouts for *Gladiators* were held at Woolwich Barracks in London. There were fifty guys there, and I had to be one of the youngest at 21 years old. My best friend, Tom (better known to wrestling fans as Bram), was there too, as was Daniel Singh, another wrestling buddy who went on to star in season two as 'Warrior'. I was intimidated; I was seeing all these guys that I had seen in muscle magazines, on TV shows and in professional sports and just thought I had a snowball's chance in hell of getting picked. But then this great sense of relaxation washed over me; I realised I had no expectations but I also had nothing to lose, so I was going to let it all go and push myself to the limit. They had these brutal assault course things set up, all designed to see how much you could bring it in one minute or two minutes.

I was holding my own, then they suddenly shouted out, "Will the following 25 people stand up..."

They read out the names, and I wasn't on the list. I feared the worst – but then they suddenly said to those 25, "Thanks for coming but you haven't been successful, go home."

Just like that, I now had a more than 1 in 5 chance (they wanted six guys) and they put us to another assault course that included chin-ups, throwing a heavy ball, sprinting and some other stuff I can't remember. I stepped up, already spent, and said to myself, "Nothing to lose." I pushed myself as hard in 90 seconds as I ever have in my life, and made it in the top five times.

One minute later, I knew I had to puke. I also knew that if the producers saw me puking I wouldn't get the gig.

I shot a look to Dan while I walked to the big shutter doors that led outside, and he immediately followed me. I walked behind an air conditioning unit and unloaded. Dan watched the door for me. I'll never forget that. I'll also never forget how great I felt knowing that I had it in me to push myself to the absolute limit when I needed to. This principle can be applied every day when you train, and if it is, it will take you places you never thought possible.

Mentally concentrating on the muscle that you're intending to stimulate plays a big role in maximising the effectiveness of these exercises. This is part of what is often referred to as "The Mind-Muscle Connection." Now before you start rolling your eyes and saying "a movement is a movement", there is research to support this. Bret Contreras aka 'The Glute Guy' (bretcontreras.com) and Brad Schoenfeld of *lookgreatnaked.com* stated, "*Simply concentrating on the target musculature resulted (according to EMG research) in greater activation of this muscle.*" Not enough for you?

Arnold Schwarzenegger is the most famous supporter of the theory. On top of that, I'm here to tell you that it works, and that's what I promised from this book, I'd tell you what works for me and others. When I was about sixteen, I was frustrated at the lack of width I had in my upper body; my chest was doing well and my other areas were starting to come through but I just didn't have that V-shaped torso. I read about Arnold's love for wide-grip chin-ups and started doing them under his guideline of 'as many sets as needed to reach a total of 50 reps'. While my strength increased and my biceps actually improved, I was still not seeing the back development. Then I started really thinking about engaging the lats (latissimus dorsi) during each rep, and within a couple of weeks I could see obvious improvement in the shape of my upper body, because I was intentionally placing as much stimulation as possible on the lats for the move. Always remember this technique when executing isolation exercises; imagine your body as a machine with each muscle having its own on/off switch. Try not to engage any other muscle except the one that you are trying to hit with the exercise; you'll be amazed at the difference in pump and stimulation you feel in the muscle. More importantly, you'll see results faster.

Get a Grip

As I alluded to earlier, we will look to pinpoint not only certain muscles, but specific areas of the muscle. There are different ways to do this; sometimes there are specific exercises, but often it can simply be a case of varying the grip you use. Good examples of this are using a reverse grip for bench press, which always really squeezed my middle pecs and helps define the line down the middle as well as my upper pecs, which is a problem area for me as I have very prominent collar bones. For the back, changing the grip is a possibility on virtually all pulling or rowing movements, which can change the area that receives the most stimulation. For example, doing rows, pulldowns or chins with a supinated grip (palms facing up) puts more emphasis on the lower lats, while a pronated grip (palms down) hits more of the upper back and a neutral grip (palms facing inwards) hits more of the middle back. Any time you feel an area is lagging behind, or you're just looking to keep your body guessing, it can be as simple as switching up your grip.

Look Good – Feel Good – Train Hard

Don't underestimate the importance of how you look while you're training. I'm not ashamed to admit it; I have a better workout when I'm wearing gym clothes that make me look good, when I have a tan, I'm well-groomed and clean shaven. If you're training properly, you'll be looking at yourself in the mirror a lot during your workout; in fact, probably more than any other time of the day. Granted, most of the time it is to make sure you maintain good form and technique, but you should also be monitoring your progress. This isn't a lottery; you don't just train, eat your food, take your supplements then take your clothes off in the summer and see what happened. You monitor your progress every day, so you can see what is working and what is not. When you see results it should motivate you.

So if you're looking at yourself in the mirror for minutes or even hours at a time while you're in the gym, and you need to be motivated to keep pushing yourself, it's just common sense to make sure you are happy with how you look while you're in there. It boils down to giving yourself the best possible chance for success. If having untidy hair or wearing unflattering clothes affects your motivation by even 1%, you should avoid it.

Gear Up

"A bad workman blames his tools", but a workman who goes to work with no tools is a dumbass.

If you're planning to train seriously, you will most likely benefit from the following pieces of gym gear:

Lifting belt – This provides support for the lower back which is very vulnerable, particularly during squats and deadlifts. While I believe that you shouldn't use a lifting belt all the time, and your lower back needs to be challenged and conditioned, there are times when the support is necessary and the additional confidence boost from the belt can help you push yourself.

Gloves – While I have never used gloves (I like to have conditioned callouses on my palms and have good grip strength) I realise that some people don't want rough calloused hands and may prefer to use gloves.

Knee wraps – I have always wrapped my knees when I squat. Just some basic compression seems to make a lot of difference for me, even if it's just mentally. Just like with lower back support, I try to leave my knees free most of the time to condition the connective tissue. But with heavy lifts, safety and support is key.

Lifting straps – A lot of people like to use straps to aid their grip strength and allow them to lift more weight. They're affordable and don't take up much space in your gym bag.

Gym bag – I'm talking specifically about the gym bag you take on to the gym floor with you, not the bag you may leave in the locker room. I see some guys bring their big duffel bag in to the weight room with them and I think that's a bit of a faux pas. It's too big. I have my belt, towel, knee wraps and bottle in a small drawstring gym bag that doesn't take up much space at all. If you need more stuff, use a big bag but leave it in the locker room, and just bring the things you immediately need with you on to the gym floor in a smaller bag.

How to build a workout

Give a man a fish and you feed him for a day; teach him to fish and you feed him for a lifetime – Maimonides

I want this book to put you in a position that it took me and so many others years of reading, listening, trial and error to get to. Many of you reading this will already have experience and knowledge under your belt, but for less experienced folk and even for the gym rats, I hope this section will simplify the process of constructing an effective workout.

It's really easy to find a workout in a magazine and follow it to the letter and number. I've done it, and it was fun and helpful early on. From time to time, I'll still flip through a magazine looking for a workout if I'm stuck in a rut or struggling to think. However, if you want the kind of body that can *put you in the magazine* instead of just reading it, you need to develop the knowledge of how to construct your own workouts, based on your goals and development, which are ever-changing.

There are three things we're going for when we look to improve our physique:

Lean Mass – acquiring the muscle itself is first priority. How much mass you want is entirely up to you. This applies to all physique goals, male or female.

Definition – defining the entire shape of the muscle so it's visible in its entirety. Achieving visible striations (lines of muscle fibres) and sharp insertions (where the muscle meets the joint, e.g. the biceps and triceps at the elbow).

Separation – Working on the areas where muscles meet and defining it so the lines of separation are visible and give you a chiselled look. Good examples include the line between the quadriceps and hamstrings in the thighs, and the upper body trifecta of the upper pectorals in the chest, the trapezius and the deltoids (shoulders).

Storm the compound(s)

Like I pointed out in *10 To Remember*, the basic process of building the body you want, regardless of size, is basic sculpting: acquire the base material, then chisel it down to the shape and proportions you want. The best way to get the base material is with **compound exercises.**

A compound exercise is a move that requires multiple muscle groups and joints to work at the same time. They are absolutely vital to developing not only the larger muscle groups, but the smaller stabiliser muscles, resulting in a base on which you can build and shape the body you want with **isolation exercises** for individual muscles. Compound moves also increase overall strength and the requirement of multiple muscle groups to fire at once causes an increase in Growth Hormone production, which aids muscular development and fat loss. The performance-enhancing properties of compound exercises cannot be overlooked either. Strength, stability, explosive power are just some of the benefits of multi-joint movements. That's why you see NFL players, MMA fighters, rugby players and so many other athletes banging out squats, deadlifts and bench press like there's no tomorrow. By now, you're probably saying, "OK I get it, compound exercises are important." They are VITAL. That's why I'm emphasising the point.

The definitive list of compound exercises is often debated, but the three big hitters are:

Squat – The king of all exercises hits the quadriceps, glutes, hamstrings, lower back and core.

Deadlift – This exercise is as old as time but still essential for developing the base on which to build your superstar body. The lower back (spinal erectors), hamstrings, quads, glutes, traps and forearms all benefit from this mammoth exercise.

Bench Press – Forever seen as the icon of upper body strength, bench press primarily hits chest (pectoralis major) but also shoulders (front deltoids) and triceps.

My list also includes wide-grip pull-ups, unquestionably my exercise of choice. For me, you need to push and pull to get complete strength and mass. Wide pull-ups engage the back, especially the lats (latissimus dorsi) but also engage the biceps in a big way, your forearms and grip strength benefit from hanging, and exponentially improve as you increase in muscle mass.

I don't think there is a better exercise you can do to achieve the classic V-shape of wide shoulders and slim waist than wide pull-ups.

Remembering that this chapter is about how to construct an effective workout, I'll take this compound principle a step further, showing what I believe to be the fundamental or compound move for each major body part. Keeping with the basic sculpting principle of adding the material, then chiselling it down and shaping it, the tried and tested approach is to build your workout around a basic fundamental or compound move, then move on to isolation exercises to further engage and stimulate the muscle fibres and induce definition, separation and quality. Here are my fundamental exercises from head to toe:

Traps – Shrugs, with either a barbell or heavy dumbbells.

Shoulders – Military press or heavy dumbbell press.

Chest – Bench press.

Biceps – Barbell curl, hammer curl.

Triceps – Skullcrushers with barbell or dumbbells.

Forearms – Barbell wrist curl.

Abdominals – Crunch, sit-up, plank.

Lower back – Deadlift.

Quadriceps/Glutes – Squat.

Hamstrings – Lying leg curl.

Calves – Calf raise.

Your form when executing compound movements should be strict, as it should be with every exercise to prevent injury and increase effectiveness. But with compound moves, you're allowed a little wiggle room when it comes to cheating (the *cheating principle* is described in the training principles chapter). The whole point of compound moves is that they target a large number of muscle groups, even though they will still usually favour one in particular. It's OK to use your whole body to get the most out of the lift, that's the intention. Almost all compound moves will require some engagement of the core, so if you're not currently using compound moves in your workouts, don't be surprised to see an improvement in your midsection.

Ladies, these moves are for you too. Some of the best female bodies I've ever seen belong to ladies who train with a range of compound moves (see *Brooke Adams*). Men are guilty of it too, but in my experience, a lot of females shy away from moves like squats and deadlifts as they think they are too 'manly' and will make them too 'butch'. Nothing could be further from the truth. A heavily muscled look is generally difficult for women to achieve as they don't have enough testosterone. In addition, nobody said you have to lift heavy. These moves can be incredibly effective for overall fat loss and improving all-round shape when used with higher reps and lighter weight for women.

Divide and Conquer

So we build the foundation (*mass*) with the compound movements; or to use my preferred analogy, we assemble the big lump of clay. Then we shape and sculpt the clay using **isolation exercises** to pinpoint certain muscles, or even specific areas of one muscle. This achieves the previously mentioned definition and separation. There are a huge number of isolation exercises that hit individual muscles or certain areas of muscles, and as many as possible will be listed in the exercise directory. Typically, an isolation exercise should be a move you can complete using as close to 100% of the target muscle as possible to complete the move; for example, a concentration curl targeting the bicep or a seated leg extension for the quads.

Time to Split

Before you construct your workouts, you have to decide which body parts you are going to train on which days. This is known as your *training split*. This method has been tried and tested for years. With the recent increase in popularity of CrossFit and functional training, there has been somewhat of a movement to suggest that you shouldn't utilise a training split, and instead train more holistically, or train your whole body. While I agree that sometimes it's great to train your whole body and work on your functionality, the fact is that if your goal is to improve the way you look, then you're going to need to spend a dedicated amount of time stimulating one or two target areas at a time to shock them to change. I don't know a single person who trains their whole body every day and looks remotely as good as someone who divides up their body parts. The Split System was first articulated by the legendary Joe Weider, but I dare say was already in use by many guys back in those days. Joe Weider, The *Weider Principles* and other training principles are described in detail in the *Training Principles* section.

Your training split should be based on your goals, and there are popular splits that have been proven to be effective. But in reality you are free to divide up the body parts you train however you like. I make a point to change my split from time to time, or change the order of my split, but typically I use a four-day split that looks like this:

Day 1: Chest and calves

Day 2: Back and hamstrings

Day 3: Quads and shoulders (I train traps with shoulders)

Day 4: Biceps and triceps (I train forearms with arms)

I work on a four-day split because then it gives me a couple of days (I train six days per week) to train whatever I feel needs work (calves!) or to do something different in the gym like power training or circuit training. I enjoy having that freedom and look forward to hitting all my body parts for the week and rewarding myself with some fun or interesting stuff on my 'open' days. I train hamstrings with back because it's important to train your lower back which can often be neglected, and when you train your lower back it ties in with the hamstrings as you have to maintain stiff legs for certain lifts which is already stimulating the hamstrings.

Beginner's Split – Total body: If you're a complete beginner, you might consider training your entire body in a single workout, with just one exercise per body part to avoid over-training. This is because in the early days of training, the primary response from the body is via the nervous system; teaching the body first to activate required muscle fibres before actively breaking them down to build back stronger (hypertrophy).

Novice Split – Push/Pull: For people who have started to get used to the processes involved in weight training, a natural progression is to do a Push/Pull split. It usually looks like this:

Day 1: Push exercises (e.g. squat, bench press, military press, leg press, calf raise, tricep pressdown etc.)

Day 2: Pull exercises (e.g. pull-ups, bicep curl, lying leg curl, barbell row)

Day 3: Rest

Alternative Novice Split – Upper/Lower body: Same principle as Push/Pull, but with a split between all upper body exercises and lower body exercises.

Day 1: Upper body

Day 2: Lower body

Day 3: Rest

Intermediate Split – Three-Day Split: As you get more conditioned you start to up the intensity, adding more sets and exercises per body part but dividing your body parts between three training days. For example:

Day 1: Chest/shoulders/triceps

Day 2: Back/biceps/core

Day 3: Quads/hamstrings/calves

Experienced Split – Dedicating a workout to either one major body part or one major body part with one minor body part. For example:

Day 1: Chest/calves

Day 2: Back/biceps

Day 3: Quads/forearms

Day 4: Hamstrings/shoulders

Advanced Split – I like adding a fifth day to dedicate to problem parts and a priority area. This is for people who are going to go and train a body part with such intensity that it will need days to recover, which is why the body parts are divided over five days. For example:

Day 1: Chest
Day 2: Back
Day 3: Legs (quads, hamstrings)
Day 4: Biceps/triceps
Day 5: Traps/forearms/calves plus any priority bodypart.

Very Advanced **Double Split** – Pioneered by the one and only Arnold, "The Oak" dedicated his whole life to building the ultimate physique, and concluded that with adequate nutrition and rest, he could recover quickly enough to hit each body part every other day for six days, taking one day to completely rest. Only attempt this once you have got used to a wide range of exercises for every body part, and you are willing to be on point with your diet, supplementation, rest and recovery techniques. If not, you will end up *over-training*, and will actually hinder your progress. For example:

Days 1, 3, 5:
AM: Chest/back
PM: Quads/hamstrings/abs

Days 2, 4, 6:
AM: Shoulders/biceps/triceps
PM: Calves/abs

Training Principles and Techniques

A vital part of building an effective workout is understanding what principle you are going to apply. This is without doubt one of the most overlooked elements from novices or people who are deferring to personal trainers. I believe that to really get the superstar body you want, you have to be tuned in mentally to what you're doing in the gym and more importantly, why you are doing it.

The Weider Principles

Most of the training principles we use today were defined by the father of bodybuilding Joe Weider. I remember when I first read these principles at about 15 years old and thinking, "I was kind of thinking that anyway," when I read a few of the principles like *instinctive training* and *muscle priority*. This was a huge motivator because now I understood that I was on the right track, and the guy that made fitness a worldwide business was confirming it. Read these principles, refer back to them as often as you need to, and apply one or several at a time to your workouts once you have them mapped out.

Cycle Training – Dedicate periods of your training year to specific goals e.g. mass, definition, strength, explosive power. This technique helps you stay on track; so many guys I know go through short phases of wanting to get bigger, then get frustrated that they're soft and then suddenly decide they want to be cut. It also adds variety and gives you something to look forward to. Changing the stresses on your muscle fibres for extended periods also allows better recovery and reduces injury risk.

Muscle Confusion – We've already discussed the importance of shocking the body, stimulating it to adapt. The muscle confusion principle is the embodiment of this point. Always keep the body guessing, by changing things up. This doesn't necessarily mean you have to change your entire workout; it can simply mean changing a few variables: number of sets, number of reps, the order of the exercise in your current routine, the length of your rest period in between sets and of course, applying a different training principle! Always strive to do at least one thing differently from your previous workout.

Instinctive Training – As you move forward, if you are mentally tuned in to what you're doing and how it feels, you will start to instinctively feel that there are things you should do. Trust those instincts and do them! You may have four sets of bench press in your plan, but you may think, "I need to hit one more set to fully pump and exhaust my chest." Lie down and bang out another set! I even apply this to my diet. Conventional advice always says to avoid carbohydrates late at night, but occasionally after a really heavy or intense session, 11pm rolls around and I want to devour some carbs, and sometimes I'll do it because I trust my instinct. And often I'll wake up the next day and my muscles have a fuller, pumped-up look and my abs will be showing more prominently! Trust your instincts, everybody and *every body* is different and if something feels right, try it.

Eclectic Training – This ties in with Muscle Confusion. Basically it means apply a diverse selection of variables (sets, reps, exercises etc) to your workouts. Remember to include both multi-joint (compound) and single-joint (isolation) exercises.

Progressive Overload – This is perhaps the most well-known of the Weider principles. As the name suggests, the idea is that you have to increase the stimulation on your muscle every time you train in order to progressively make gains. This can mean adding weight, adding sets, adding exercises, shortening rest periods or any number of intensity techniques. Just be sure that you subjected your body to a little more work than you did in the last workout.

Muscle Priority – This principle refers to you identifying and exposing your weak points. Self-awareness is key. Basically, hit your weakest body part first when you are fresh and can train more intensely. For example, if I'm training calves, I always have to train them first, because they are a weak point for me. If I'm fresh, I can use drop sets, partial reps and other techniques to make sure I did my best to spur growth.

Pyramid Training – A commonly used approach, Pyramid Training means to go from lighter to heavier weight during each exercise, gradually increasing with each set. You can reverse this process, and start heavy then move down in weight and increase reps, this is called a *Reverse Pyramid*. I actually incorporated reverse pyramid training a lot in my early years of training, as I wanted to increase my strength, so I wanted to move as much weight as I could which meant being fresh.

Peak Contraction – This is a great way to add definition and separation as well as muscle control. Squeeze the contracted muscle at the end point or 'top' of the rep. Aim to hold the fully contracted and squeezed position for about two seconds.

Iso-Tension – This principle works in the same way as Peak Contraction, increasing definition, separation and especially adding muscle control. In between sets, flex and hold your muscles, specifically the ones being worked, and hold for a few seconds. Get into this habit, you will get a harder, more chiselled look.

Continuous Tension – Control the positive (flex) portion of the movement and the negative (extension) portion by repping more slowly and avoiding using momentum. This maintains constant tension in the muscle fibres which subsequently tears more fibres and means you make better gains.

Holistic Training – Similar to Eclectic Training, Holistic Training means using numerous techniques to stimulate your body and muscle fibres and not just always approaching everything with the same style. For example, sometimes use a faster rep speed, sometimes go for higher reps and give your joints a rest and stimulate your slow-twitch muscle fibres. Keep it varied to enjoy your body and realise its potential.

Flushing Training – This is a great example of a technique most people use today but may not realise it has a name. Flushing means to train one body part fully with multiple exercises before you move on to another. The reason you do this is to maximise blood flow and nutrient delivery to the area and give the best chance for growth and improvement.

Isolation Training – Already discussed in detail, this pertains to working individual muscles while minimising the use of other muscle groups.

Supersets – Perform two exercises back-to-back with no rest period in between. This is a great way to train with limited time and can be used for the same or different muscle groups. I love to train with supersets; the slight variation can be enough to feel different and get more out of the workout. For example, you may only be able to complete 10 full reps of barbell bicep curls, but if you superset them with dumbbell concentration curls, you may be able to get an additional 6 or 7 reps after completing the 10 barbell curls.

Tri-Sets – The same principle as supersets but with three exercises back-to-back.

Giant Sets – Once again the same principle as supersets, but with four or more exercises performed back-to-back.

Burns – Once you've reached the point where you can't fully lift the weight any more, lift it as much as you can over and over again even if you're only moving the weight a few inches. This is a great way to finish off a workout and tear as many fibres as possible.

Partial Reps – You actually use Partial Reps during Burns but by necessity. You can also deliberately use partial reps – the bottom portion, middle or top portion of a movement to focus on a weaker point or to emphasise stimulation to a specific area of a muscle. For example, if you want a more defined bicep 'peak' then using partial reps of just the top portion of the movement can help.

Cheating – The cheating principle should be used with caution. This is not a free pass to use bad form. Cheating means to use a small amount of momentum (a little swing) to complete extra reps after reaching failure with strict form. This should only be used by experienced trainers. Arnold Schwarzenegger believed in the cheating principle especially to build his iconic biceps.

Forced Reps – In the same family as cheating, forced reps is using a training partner or spotter to help you through sticking points at the end of a set to achieve maximum stimulation. Your spotter should only use the amount of force needed to get you through the move, so the majority of the work stays with you.

Drop Sets – One of my personal favourites, Drop Sets means reaching the point of failure at a certain weight, then quickly reducing the weight and continuing with lighter weight until failure, then descending again. This will burn you out and really pump you up. If training alone, dumbbells or machines is the best way to utilise this technique.

Pre-Exhaustion – This is the opposite approach to typically starting a workout with compound multi-joint movements then progressing to isolation exercises. With the pre-exhaust method, you use single-joint isolation moves first then finish with multi-joint moves. This is useful if you have a weak area of a muscle, or if the other muscles used in multi-joint movements burn out before the target muscle. I used pre-exhaustion to improve my shoulders when they were a major weak point. My triceps would take a lot of the brunt of heavy presses due to my long arms and they would burn out before I really felt my deltoids had been stimulated. So I started doing lateral raises, front raises for the front deltoids and bent over laterals for the rear deltoids before I did any pressing movements. I soon had a more rounded and balanced deltoid muscle.

Negatives – The upward part of the exercise is called the positive portion, while the descending part is called the negative. Typically, the focus is on the positive portion, but deliberately slowing and resisting on the negative portion stimulates the muscle in a completely different way. Often people will use a spotter to aid on the positive portion so they can do the negative as slowly as possible, which really burns.

Rest-Pause – This is another technique I used regularly before I ever read about it as a defined technique. Work to the point of failure, take a few seconds or more, then squeeze out one or two more reps as part of the same set.

Other Principles

21's – Most commonly used for biceps, this technique requires you to perform seven partial reps of the lower third of a movement, seven partial reps of the middle third of the movement then seven partial reps of the upper third, back-to-back. You can apply the technique to several different exercises to change things up.

Isometric Tension – There are two types of contraction: Isotonic (with movement) and Isometric (stationary). Most exercises are Isotonic, but burning out your muscles fibres with Isometric moves can really add definition and separation. I regularly use isometrics for shoulders, holding a pair of dumbbells out at my sides for as long as possible. When I first went to wrestling school, we were all subjected to the dreaded 'wall chair', having to hold a partial squat against a wall so your thighs are parallel to the floor for as long as possible. Planks have become a popular core movement, and are another great example of isometric exercise. Isometrics can be very beneficial to balance, so if you want to improve your performance in your sport (or in the bedroom) isometrics should be considered.

Blood Flow Restriction training (BFR) – BFR is a relatively new, cutting-edge technique that I have started using for my arms and legs. Basically, you restrict the blood flow with a band or wrap on the veins, not the arteries and perform a set of high reps. The restriction causes cell swelling. When your cells swell, they restructure themselves and get bigger, meaning bigger muscle cells. Also, lactic acid gets trapped in the muscle. Now most people think of lactic acid as a negative thing, which it is when it comes to cardio, but LA is actually anabolic (muscle building) and the presence of it aids protein synthesis (if you're interested in this, look it up, it's too wordy for me; I don't want to bore you to tears with science). I find that doing a short BFR workout on a non-arm day allows me to have a fuller, more pumped bicep and tricep all the time without over-training them. It's an advanced technique, so please proceed with caution and read up more on BFR. There are some great articles at bodybuilding.com.

Superstar Spotlight – Daniel Singh

Through the years of training for various different disciplines, I've always had to adapt in order to suffice the demands my body required. Whether it be bodybuilding, professional wrestling, MMA or purely for aesthetics, I used to train sports specifically meaning that other elements of my physique, either for function or aesthetics began to lag.

It was with that in mind that I opted to perform a method of training that catered for every element of my needs and I came up with TUT (Time Under Tension) Power Training.

Theoretically it's a combination of power training on the compound movements, which I believe is a necessity to really build density and efficient core strength, in combination with isolation bodybuilding movements to really stimulate the fibres and contribute maximal growth. It's with this method in mind that I find that I am never a million miles away from being able to adapt more towards being in shape for a photo shoot, gearing towards a maximal lift or being functionally able in order to prepare for an upcoming fight.

A typical workout would be as follows:

Back Day
Compound movement – Deadlifts 3 sets – 5, 3 , 3
Pendlay rows – 3 sets – 5, 5, 5
Kayak rows – 3 sets TUT – 8, 8, 8

Straight arm pull-overs (rope), hip hinge 90 degree, slight elevation ¾ extend plus forced contraction 3 sets of 8 on each motion.
HIIT

So as you can see the initial movements would cover the core foundations to develop power/density and thickness whilst the remaining movements are more so to develop over all fibres and aid general fitness and conditioning. This is how I incorporate all of my workouts to ensure I achieve fundamental strength in squats, bench, deadlifts, cleans etc, mainly Olympic lifts to complement aesthetics. I've found this style of training allows versatility along with longevity, which is hugely important to maintaining a decent duration shelf life for any athlete, preventing injury.

Daniel Singh is an actor, former television personality as 'Warrior' on Gladiators, MMA fighter and owner of Gladiator Nutrition Supplement Store. You may recognise Dan as the face of 'Big Scary Gym' for the energie fitness clubs commercials.
Twitter and Instagram: @DanWarriorSingh
Facebook: Gladiator Nutrition Durham

Build your Workout Reference Table

I've devised this table so you can use it as a quick reference guide as you're planning your workouts. Notice that I've used the word *recommended* when it comes to set/rep range and training principles for certain body parts. This is because *there are no rules!* You can do as few or as many reps as you want, you can apply any principle you want, but in my experience the recommended ones are the ones that work most effectively.

Couple of housekeeping points: Work Sets refers to sets where you're going 100%. You should always perform some warm-up sets with a light weight to get heat and blood into your muscles and joints. I perform at least one warm-up set of every exercise I do, sometimes more than one, especially if the area is prone to strains, like hamstrings or back. For the sake of space saving, I have abbreviated Barbell to 'BB' and Dumbbell to 'DB'. Check out www.EXRX.net for moving GIFS of almost every resistance exercise out there, or link to it through www.superstarbodybook.com

Body Part	Compound Exercise	Isolation Exercises	Recommended Set/ Rep Range	Recommended Training Principles
Chest	Bench Press	*Upper Pecs:* Incline Press, Incline DB Press, Incline DB Flyes, Incline Cable Flyes *Lower Pecs:* Decline Bench Press, Decline DB Bench Press, Decline DB Flyes, Reverse-Grip Bench Press, Dips *Middle Pecs:* DB Flyes, Pec Deck Flyes, Cable Flyes, DB Bench Press, Machine Press, Close Grip Push-Ups Outer Pecs: Wide Grip Bench Press, Extreme Range Push Up, DB/Cable/Machine Flyes w/ partial range.	4-5 exercises, 4-5 work sets per exercise, typically in the 6-12 rep range, depending on your goals.	Flushing Drop Sets Burns Rest-Pause 21s Supersets

Body Part	Compound Exercise	Isolation Exercises	Recommended Set / Rep Range	Recommended Training Principles
Back (Upper/Lats)	Wide Grip Chin Up	*Upper Back:* Behind-Neck Pulldown, Standing Wide-Grip Cable Row *Middle Back:* Barbell Row, DB Row, Cable Row, Machine Row, Lat Pulldown. Straight-Arm Pulldown, DB Pullover Lower Lats: Reverse-grip Pulldown, Reverse-grip BB Row, Reverse-grip Cable Row	4-5 exercises, 4-5 work sets per exercise, typically in the 6-12 rep range, depending on your goals.	Supersets Burns Cheating Forced Reps Isometric Training
Lower Back	Deadlift	Good Mornings Back Extensions Back Extension Machine	3-4 exercises, 3-4 work sets per exercise. Rep range 8-15 (excluding Deadlift which can be heavy with lower reps)	Iso-tension Rest-Pause Isometric Training Partial Reps

Body Part	Compound Exercise	Isolation Exercises	Recommended Set/ Rep Range	Recommended Training Principles
Shoulders	Barbell Military Press	*Front Deltoids:* Behind-the-neck Press, Front Lateral Raise (BB, DB & Cable), DB Press, Arnold Press, Smith Machine Press. Upright Rows (BB & Cable) *Middle Deltoids:* Machine Press, Lateral Raise (DB & Cable), Lying DB Side Laterals *Rotator Cuff:* Internal Rotations (DB & Resistance Band), External Rotations, DB Cuban Rotations (DB & BB) *Rear Deltoids:* Reverse Pec Deck, Cable Reverse Flye, Best Over Lateral Raise (standing, seated, incline bench, face-supported), Cable Face Pull (Rope)	4-5 exercises, 4-5 work sets per exercise, typically in the 6-12 rep range, depending on your goals.	Pre-exhaust Flushing Supersets, Tri-sets, Giant Sets Rest-Pause Continuous Tension Isometric Training Drop Sets

Body Part	Compound Exercise	Isolation Exercises	Recommended Set/ Rep Range	Recommended Training Principles
Quadriceps	Squat Deadlift	Leg Extensions, Sissy Squats, Leg Press, Lunges (BB & DB) Hack Squat, Box Jumps *Outer Quads*: Narrow-stance squat/press *Inner Quads*: Wide-stance squat/press	5-6 exercises; at least 5 work sets per exercise. Rep range should be higher than other muscles; staying in the 8-20 rep range.	Pyramid Training Muscle Confusion Rest-Pause Peak Contraction Blood Flow Restriction Training (BFR)

Body Part	Compound Exercise	Isolation Exercises	Recommended Set/ Rep Range	Recommended Training Principles
Hamstrings	Deadlift, Stiff-legged Deadlift	Lying Leg Curl, Good Mornings, DB Romanian Deadlift, Standing Leg Curl Machine, Standing Cable Leg Curl, Glute/Ham Raise, Exercise Ball Leg Curl	3-4 exercises; 4-5 work sets per exercise, rep range should be in the 8-15 range.	Isolation Training Continuous Tension Peak Contraction Flushing Blood Flow Restriction Training (BFR)
Calves	Standing Calf Raise	Donkey Calf Raise, Seated Calf Raise, Calf Machine, Modified Farmer's Walk (DB, on toes)	3-4 exercises; 4-5 work sets per exercise, rep range should be in the 8-15 range.	Drop Sets Flushing Peak Contraction BFR

Body Part	Compound Exercise	Isolation Exercises	Recommended Set/Rep Range	Recommended Training Principles
Biceps	Barbell Curl	DB Concentration Curl, Incline DB Curl, Preacher Curl (BB, DB, Cable, EZ Bar or Machine) Cable Curl (Lying or Standing) Machine Curl, EZ Bar Curl. *Forearm emphasis:* Hammer Curl (DB or Cable with rope) Reverse-grip Curl (EZ Bar or BB)	3-5 exercises; 3-5 work sets depending on rep range and intensity. I tend to stay in the 6-12 rep range.	Peak Contraction 21's BFR Cheating Drop Sets Negatives
Triceps	Skull Crushers (aka French Press, with EZ Bar or Barbell) Close-Grip Bench Press	DB Overhead Extension, Kickbacks (DB or Cable), Lying DB Cross-body Extension, Bodyweight Tricep Extension (Bar or Suspension Cables) Bench Dip, Dips (Bodyweight or Machine) Bodyweight Tricep Extension	3-5 exercises; 3-5 work sets depending on rep range and intensity. I tend to stay in the 6-12 rep range.	Peak Contraction 21's BFR Pre-exhaust
Forearms	Barbell Wrist Curl	Wrist Curl (DB, Cable, Machine) Isometric grips w/plates, Hammer Curl, Reverse-grip Curl (BB or EZ Bar)	2-3 exercises, 3-5 work sets. Forearms need heavy weight to be stimulated so typically 6-10 rep range works well.	Pyramid Training Drop Sets Continuous Tension

Body Part	Compound Exercise	Isolation Exercises	Recommended Set/ Rep Range	Recommended Training Principles
Trapezius (Traps)	Barbell Shrug	DB Shrug, Cable Shrug, Shrug Machine, Shrug using Calf Raise Machine, Upright Rows (BB or EZ Bar)	2-3 exercises, 4-6 work sets. Traps respond to heavy weight, so rep range can be as little as 4, but up to 12 or 15.	Pyramid training Drop Sets
Abdominals & Core	Sit-up	*Upper Abs Focus:* Crunch, Ball Crunch, Cable Crunch, Machine Crunch, Decline Sit-Up, Roman Chair Sit-Up, Plank. *Lower Abs Focus:* Reverse Crunch, Ab Wheel Rollout, Ball Pull-Ins, Hanging Leg Raise, Jackknife Sit-Up *Obliques Focus:* Standing Twist, Oblique Crunches, Side Bends, Lying Side Raises, Elbow-to-Knee Crunch, Cable Side Bends, Cable Woodchop.	The muscles of the abdomen are primarily made up of fast-twitch fibres. Treat them like any other muscle; 4-5 exercises, 3-4 work sets, 8-12 rep range.	Supersets, Tri-sets, Giant Sets Continuous Tension Negatives Rest-Pause Burns

Body Part	Compound Exercise	Isolation Exercises	Recommended Set/ Rep Range	Recommended Training Principles
Glutes & Inner/Outer Thighs	Lunges	*Glutes*: Cable Leg Kick-Back, Glutes Machine, BB Glute Bridge, Flutter Kicks Inner Thigh (Adductor): Adductor Machine, Sumo Squat, Cable Adduction. Outer Thigh (Abductor): Abductor Machine, Monster Walk, Windmills	Glutes are a large muscle, and contain a lot of fast-twitch fibres, so respond better to hypertrophic (muscle building) work; 2-3 exercises, 3-4 work sets, 8-15 rep range. Adductors and Abductors are smaller and more sensitive so generally respond to higher reps, stay in 12-20 range.	Pyramid Training Drop Sets Peak Contraction

How To Build a Workout – Summary

With this section, hopefully you now have a good template to use when it comes to constructing your workout for your goals. In my opinion, these are the fundamental steps:

1. Be honest with yourself and assess whether you are a beginner, intermediate, advanced or expert trainer.

2. Choose a training split that meets your current level.

3. Design your workouts based on the information already given, remembering the importance of compound exercises and the benefits of isolation exercises.

4. Apply the different training principles to fast-track your results.

5. Re-assess yourself about every six weeks or so and repeat the process.

Chest

There's something about a well-developed chest that commands respect. As a kid, I could see guys that had big arms and be impressed, but when I saw a guy with a great overall physique punctuated by full, square pecs it immediately captivated my imagination and I would think, "That's how I want to look."

For centuries, the chest has been an incredibly symbolic area of the body; as the location of the heart, it is an important part of the anatomy, which requires it to be well protected. People instinctively look at other humans' chests (not just women's chests, easy, tiger), which is why throughout history, military, sports teams, law enforcement and even everyday customer service employees usually wear some form of identification on their chest. Gorillas, our closest relatives along with chimpanzees, beat their chests to symbolise their strength and ability when posed with a perceived threat and display their dominance (how many times have you seen athletes do it after a win or a score?).

For men, a well-developed and symmetrical chest is a game-changer; there are always going to be guys who do endless bicep curls so their arms look good at the club in a t-shirt, or guys who obsess over abdominals so they can lift up their shirt and show a six-pack. But in my experience, many times these guys have no chest and that appealing, masculine look that they're going for isn't quite there. I can tell you from personal experience that the one thing I'm complimented on most frequently by women when it comes to physique is my chest.

For women's physiques, obviously the chest is a focal point for other reasons, but strong and lean pectoral muscles can help elevate the breasts and maintain their lift and shape, which is obviously very appealing and a desired look for many women.

Training the Chest

The pectorals (*pectoralis major and minor*) anatomically are divided into the upper (clavicular) and lower (sternal) but in my opinion, to achieve a full and lean chest you need to think of the pectorals in four sections: upper, lower, outer and middle. You can see exercises that target these specific areas in the *Build Your Workout Reference Table.* For me, the upper pecs have always been the stubborn area of my chest. I will frequently start my chest workout with Incline Press and with Incline Flyes to make sure I am fresh and can devote as much of my strength to hitting the upper pecs as possible. Mentally engaging that target area using the mind-muscle connection is very effective for targeting areas of the chest; most of the movements are very similar, they're either a press or a flye. So the style of contraction and mentally focusing on the area you wish to engage are the keys to developing the entire chest.

When targeting the *upper chest*, focus on hitting at least two or three incline movements e.g. Incline Bench Press, Incline Dumbbell Press and Incline Flyes. Focus on the contraction at the top of the movement and squeeze the upper chest together when completing each rep. Keep in mind that when you train upper chest with incline movements, you engage the front deltoids a lot, so keep that in mind when making your training split as your front deltoids will be sore after training upper chest and will need to recover also.

If you want more mass in the *lower chest*, decline presses should be first priority, whether it be with a barbell or dumbbells. As with upper pecs, focus on engaging the lower pecs, especially when completing each rep, squeezing the contraction and forcing blood to the area. Cable flyes with the cable pulley positioned up high are also great for the lower pecs. Finally, dips are a tried and tested move for lower pec development and really help separate the pecs from the ribcage, which gives that square, muscular look that really defines a good chest.

When targeting the *outer chest*, the important word is **stretch**. The largest portion of the pectorals is the outer portion that inserts at the armpit. The best way to hit this area is to ensure that you achieve the full stretch and range of motion when doing dumbbell flyes, cable flyes (mid-height pulley position) and presses with a wide or standard grip. It's important to remember that most chest exercises will hit more than one area. For example, a well-executed flye will stretch and engage the outer pecs on the negative portion and contract and squeeze the middle pecs at the top of the positive portion. But if you are adamant on specifically hitting just the outers, you can perform partial reps, avoiding the squeeze at the top of the contraction.

The key principle when looking to improve the *middle* or *inner pecs* is peak contraction. Yes, using close grip on presses will hit the inner pecs, but it will also engage the triceps a lot and in my opinion, is not enough to get the inner pecs going. As I described in the above paragraph, the squeeze at the top of most chest movements will emphasise the middle chest; and similar to outer pecs prioritising, partial reps can also be used, keeping as much resistance and stimulation on the inner pecs as possible. The most effective way to do this is with a pec deck machine or with cables. Using dumbbells for this is likely to burn out your shoulders and biceps before you get the full stimulation of the inner chest needed.

Back

Much like my point about being noticed for things besides biceps and abs before, a thick, wide back implies power, stability and strength. And guys, don't overlook the appeal of a good back; a lot of women are very attracted to a strong muscular back, it makes them feel safe, which is a big plus when analysing the male form.

Training the Back

I discovered the joy of having a good back a long time ago, but ironically, it was looking at myself from the front that got me to that point. At fifteen years old, I had started to make good strides with my chest, abs and triceps in particular. But I was frustrated with my lack of width when I stood in front of a mirror, and realised that my lats (*latissimus dorsi*) in particular were lacking.

I turned to my first point of reference for all matters at the time, Arnold, and read about his Wide-Grip chins (pull-ups) technique of performing as many sets as necessary in order to complete 50 full reps, even if it means doing sets of two or even one rep by the end, which I frequently had to in my early days. I used that technique that day and have done ever since. For me, the wide-grip pull-up is the best exercise for width, and necessary to get that v-shaped look that men in particular strive for.

For thickness, rowing exercises are going to be your best bet but nothing beats the classic bent-over barbell row. It's one of the toughest lifts ever, the strain of human force versus gravity never more apparent. You need to use a good heavy weight to get the desired results, but keep in mind that your lower back takes a great amount of pounding in this move too. Unless you really need it, try and perform this lift without a belt, and let your lower back work and develop strength to support you, but you must use perfect form, or you can do some serious damage to a very vulnerable area. Switching the grip to an underhand grip hits more of the lower lats and I always found I got a better squeeze in the middle with underhand grip.

Train the lower back almost like a separate entity: Hit it hard and give it plenty of time to recover. You need a strong lower back; please believe me when I say this. It's not the most aesthetically important muscle but it is nonetheless very important. Deadlifts, good mornings and back extensions are all part of my lower back arsenal.

Don't forget the serratus muscles, which sit between your chest and your lats. Some people train serratus with chest, I train it with back, as I feel the exercises for serratus also engage the lats. The classic exercise is the dumbbell pullover, but you can also use the pullover machine if your gym has one or my personal favourite the straight-arm pulldown, using either a bar or rope. I love this exercise; I position myself in a way that allows me to stretch my arms as far above my head as possible, almost behind my head, and then mentally focusing on engaging the lats and serratus (not the triceps) to pull the bar down keeping your arms straight to the waist. Having good serratus muscles is a way to look like you have a wider ribcage and that chiselled look when you raise your

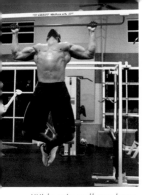

Wide grip pull ups have always been a staple of my routine.

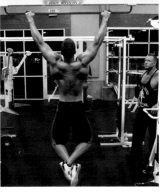

I make sure to fully hang when performing pull ups. allowing maximum effort, separation and definition.

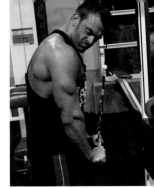

Cable pressdown

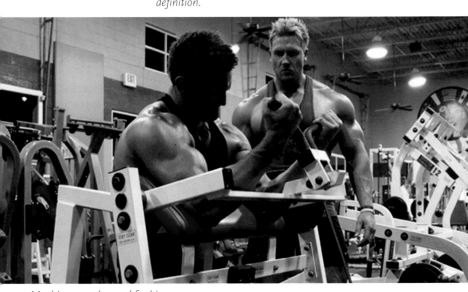

Machine preacher curl for biceps

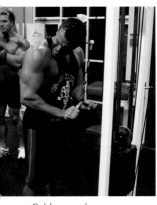

Cable pressdown

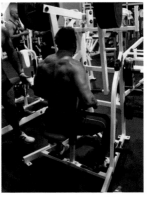

Hammer strength machine row

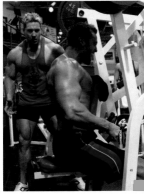

Training back with Big Rob Terry

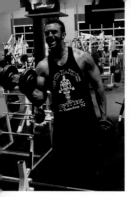

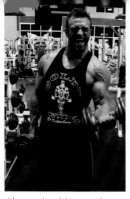

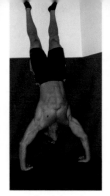

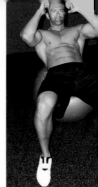

Alternating dumbbell curl

Alternating bicep curls makes you work harder with your core and forearms to complete the same number of reps. Intensity is required.

Handstand push ups against a wall are a killer. Shoulders and triceps get absolutely fried and it requires a lot of mental focus.

Swiss ball crunch

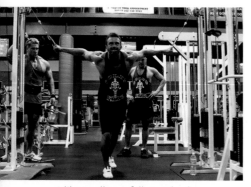

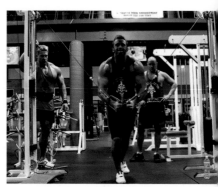

I like to allow a full stretch when I'm doing cable flyes, ensuring maximum effort for the chest.

Performing cable flyes as Rob Terry and Nigel McGuinness observe.

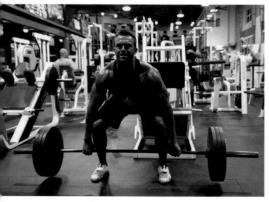

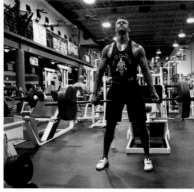

Deadlift

Deadlifting in one of my favourite gyms, Gold's Gym St Petersburg, Florida.

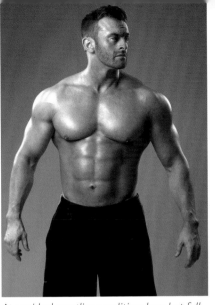

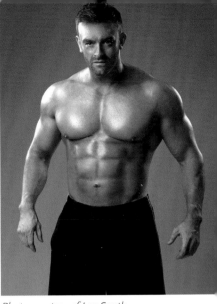

At my ideal wrestling condition; lean but full. New York City, January 2015. Photo courtesy of Lee South

Photo courtesy of Lee South

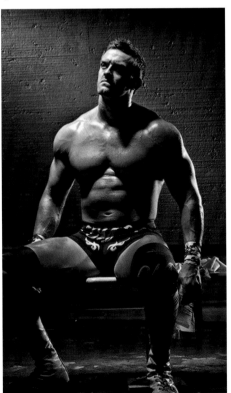

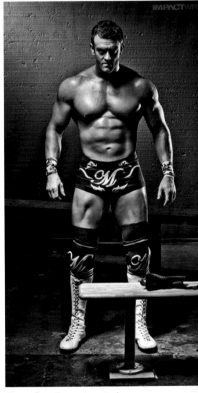

Photo courtesy of Lee South

One of my leanest periods, summer 2012. Photo courtesy of Lee South

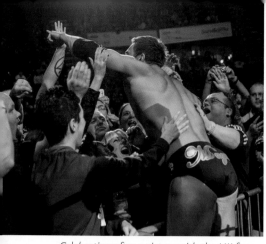

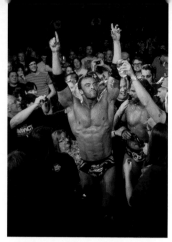

Celebrating after a victory with the UK fans who have been so good to me over the years. Photo courtesy of Tony Knox

After teaming up with James Storm, we celebrated amongst the people. I have a mouth full of beer in this picture. Photo courtesy of Tony Knox

Saluting the crowd in the Nottingham arena before my match. This is one of my favourite pictures. Photo courtesy of Tony Knox

Delivering a shoulder tackle to Kurt Angle. Photo courtesy of Lee South and TNA Entertainment LLC

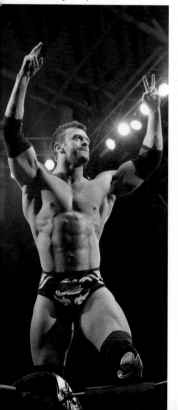

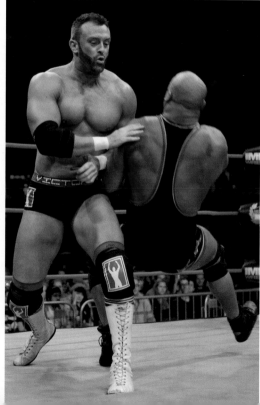

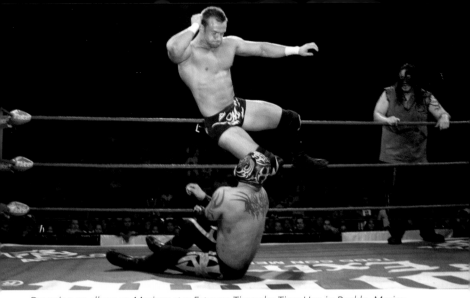

Dropping an elbow on Mexican star Extreme Tiger aka Tigre Uno in Puebla, Mexico for the AAA promotion. September 2011

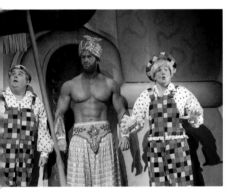

I had to stay in great condition doing two shows per day as The Genie in the Norwich Theatre Royal pantomime production of Aladdin in 2012

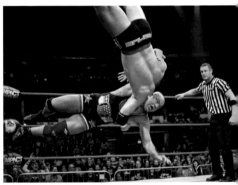

Kurt Angle giving an overhead suplex from the top rope to yours truly. Photo courtesy of Lee South and TNA Entertainment LLC

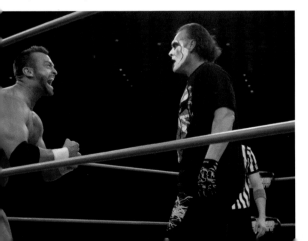

One of my proudest moments was getting to wrestle and defeat one of my heroes, Sting, at a pay per view event in San Diego, California in 2013. Photo courtesy of Lee South and TNA Entertainment LLC

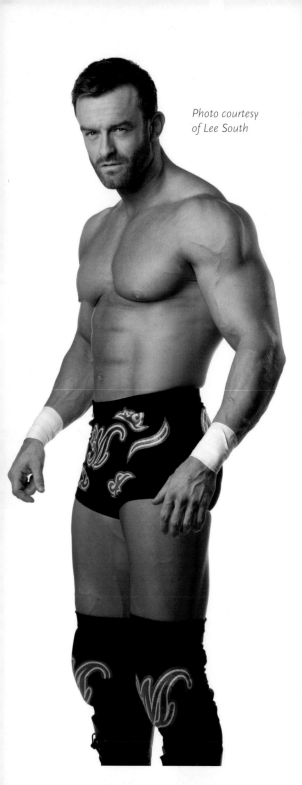

Photo courtesy
of Lee South

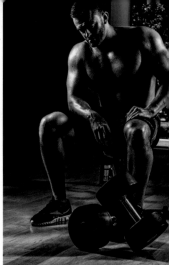

You have to look at the weight and
visualise yourself lifting it. Photo
courtesy of Lee South and TNA
Entertainment LLC

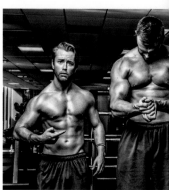

Flexing in between sets can bring
out more definition and density.
Photo courtesy of Lee South and
TNA Entertainment LLC

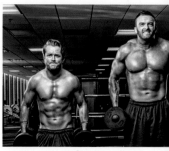

Spud was always begging to train
with me! Photo courtesy of Lee
South and TNA Entertainment LLC

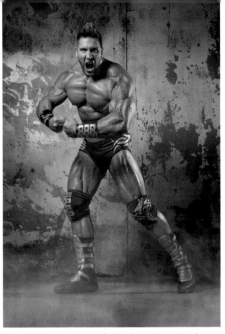

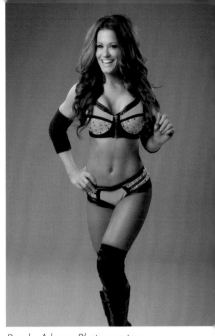

Possibly the greatest physical specimen in the history of pro wrestling; 'The Freak' Rob Terry Photo courtesy of Joey Goldsmith

Brooke Adams. Photo courtesy of Lee South and TNA Entertainment LLC

Rob Strauss aka Robbie E is fired up. Photo courtesy of Lee South and TNA Entertainment LLC

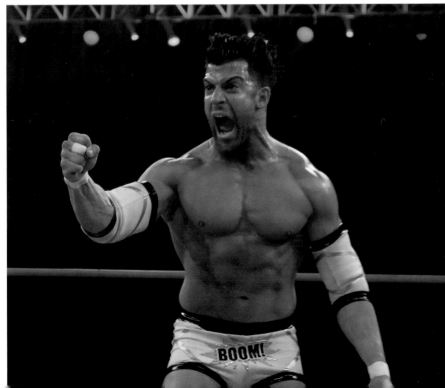

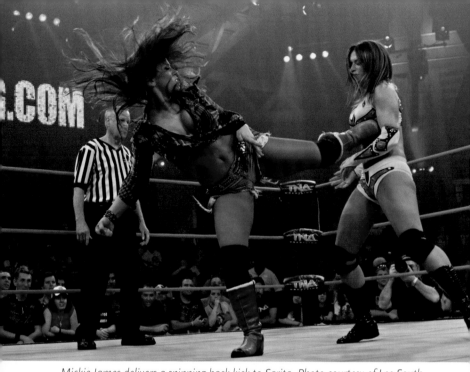

Mickie James delivers a spinning back kick to Sarita. Photo courtesy of Lee South and TNA Entertainment LLC

Kurt Angle delivers a German suplex to Bobby Lashley. Photo courtesy of Lee South and TNA Entertainment LLC

David McIntosh

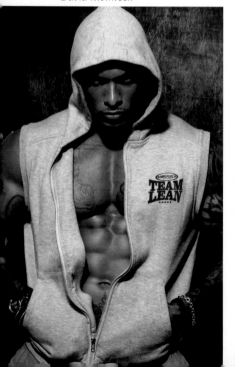

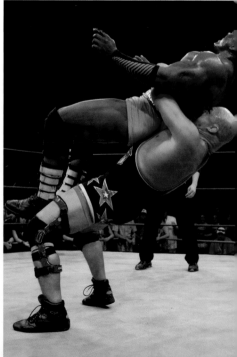

arms; that detail is one of the things that will set you apart from the average guy in the gym.

There are a ton of areas of the back and to have a complete, thick, chiselled back you need to work them all. There are so many variations of rowing movements and the pull up/down that you can't use them all in one workout. Switch things up, use different attachments on the cable like the rope or single arm pulley instead of a bar, change up your grip with underarm, neutral grip, wide and narrow grips. Add these to a workout with solid compound moves using a good weight and you're on your way to an impressive back.

Shoulders

Despite having long arms, making shoulders a tough area for me, they are possibly my favourite body part to train. There are just so many ways to pinpoint the individual heads of the *deltoid* and build mass and definition for boulder delts that always command attention. Even if you're not looking to win Mr Olympia, you should appreciate the importance of the balance that shoulders bring. For so many guys, chest and arms dominate their mindset, but great shoulders tie them together and without them, you never quite get the look you're going for. A good pair of arms really needs delts in the worst way; if you're out on the beach this summer in a sleeveless shirt and your bis and tris are full and pumped but your shirt flaps around where your deltoid is supposed to be, then you're not going to turn as many heads as you think.

Training the deltoids

Speaking of heads, there are three to concern yourself with: Front (*Anterior*), Middle (*Medial*) and Rear (*Posterior*) and that to me is the beauty of training shoulders; once you think of them as three separate areas that need to be trained equally, you will develop full, round shoulders in no time. The *front delts* undoubtedly get the most attention from your everyday trainers because they are utilised in all the pressing movements. Barbell and dumbbell press are obviously key but try to incorporate the Arnold Press and go old-school with behind-the-neck presses too. To really achieve the separation between the shoulder, chest and traps that give that chiselled look, focus on strict form with a sizeable weight and accentuate the peak contraction, squeezing the front deltoid at the top of your presses. Don't forget front raises, with a barbell, dumbbells or cables. They can really isolate the deltoid with good form and bring out the striations (little lines that ripple through the muscle). I change it up sometimes and use an EZ bar, the slight grip adjustment shifts the area of stimulation and keeps the shoulders guessing. The *middle head* of the deltoid is most effectively worked with lateral raise movements. Dumbbell laterals are a must, and remember to go heavy with them; I see so many guys doing dumbbell laterals with 30lb dumbbells when they clearly have the strength to do more, because they've got it ingrained in their head that strict form and slow reps is the most important thing with lateral raise. While strict form is always important, you have to challenge the middle head of the shoulder. Do some heavy laterals and cheat a little if you have to. Drop sets are a personal favourite of mine with laterals (dumbbell or cable) as they burn out quickly but also recover quickly so drop sets ensure that you really push them to grow and define. For *rear delts*, isolation is key; bent-over laterals using strict form, reverse pec deck is always effective, lying face down on an incline bench and doing rear delt laterals is challenging but for me, my favourite way to target and isolate the rear delt is taking a cable without any attachment and gripping the cable on the inside of where the stopper ball is, then I adjust the cable to shoulder height, step out so that my arm is completely across my chest and my rear delt is stretched, then with a straight arm, I draw the cable out and across, using just my rear deltoid. By not fighting against gravity, you can focus purely on the contraction of the rear delt, unlike with bent over laterals.

Don't neglect your rotator cuff. It's one of the smallest, strongest and most vulnerable parts of the body. And if you injure it, say bye-bye to months of training. Cuban rotations target them directly and I often pre-exhaust the rest of my shoulder training with rotator cuff training because I'm focused on injury prevention. It will improve your throwing arm too (baseball players do tons of rotator cuff training) so when you're on the beach this summer your throw will match your physique.

Quadriceps

Superstar Spotlight – Brooke Adams

There is nothing sexier than a woman who has toned/sculpted thighs and glutes. I get asked frequently what crazy over-the-top training do I do to get such toned legs and glutes. Surprisingly, I keep it pretty basic. It's not about how much weight you throw around or what exercises you can come up with. It's HOW you train. I regularly incorporate unilateral training. By isolating one limb at a time this ensures the muscles of each leg get equal work and development. So it's good to throw in a few of these exercises to your routine.

I start by doing a 10-minute warm-up on the StairMaster.

– Squats on the smith machine 3 sets for 15 reps
Be sure to hit these deep and keep your heels planted

– Reverse lunges with bench steps 3 sets for 15 reps
You can do your reverse lunges on the smith machine or by holding dumbbells.
On the bench step-ups use dumbells. You will do 15 reps per leg

– Pile Squats with weighted unilateral hip bridges 3 sets of 15/ 3 sets of 25

I do Pile squats on the smith machine. They can also be done by holding a single dumbbell between the legs or a kettle weight. I like to do these super heavy and slow.

On the hip bridges use a bench to lay your shoulders across. Lay a plate of whichever weight best suits you in the pelvic area. Be sure to squeeze on the way up.

– Bulgarian Split Squat 3 sets 20
I usually do these with dumbbells. Be sure to again drive with the heel

– Stiff Leg Dead Lifts 3 sets of 15

– Single Leg Hamstring Curls 3 sets of 25 per leg

– Single Leg extensions 3 sets of 25 per leg

– Glute cable Kickbacks 3 sets of 25 per leg
Squeeze glute hard at the top of the movement

Brooke Adams – Professional wrestler (2 x TNA Knockouts Champion), model, Miss Hawaiian Tropic Texas 2008, Hooters Viewer's Choice 2010 winner and star of* The Amazing Race *on CBS.

The first time I really made a conscious decision that I wanted to be a pro wrestler was watching Wrestlemania XV. The main event was The Rock vs Stone Cold Steve Austin and unlike the vast majority, I was rooting for The Rock. When he strutted out into the arena as the World Champion, he walked in a way that shook and flexed his quads and it was the first time I appreciated what a difference it made to a male physique (especially if you're going to wear trunks).

Quads are one of the largest muscles in the body, and play such a pivotal role in so many things like walking, running, jumping and balancing to name a few. In terms of sports performance, they are the key component in almost every facet of physical output. In terms of physique, not all people want gigantic quads that chafe and restrict movement but that doesn't mean that you should phone it in. Besides, do you know how much weight you have to shift in order to build quads like that? Trust me, you'll have plenty of time to get the size you want before you reach that level. For the ladies, I can tell you from my own personal opinion that I find athletic, toned quads with a nice smooth front sweep incredibly sexy on a woman. For some guys, quads are low on the priority list because they think, "I wear shorts or pants, nobody sees my quads." Well, genius, what happens when you get to the bedroom? If you want to wow her in your designer undies, you best have some decent quads in them.

Training the Quads

Since your quads should be subjected to a significant workload every day (walk, stand, take the stairs, people!), they are already conditioned to a lot, so to inspire growth and definition, volume is key. The general consensus is that the average overall rep range should be higher for quads, somewhere around fifteen. But that doesn't mean you shouldn't still shock-challenge them with heavy weight and lower reps. In fact, the fact that you're going for an average of fifteen reps doesn't mean you should change the weight much at all.

I remember training quads with 'The Freak' Rob Terry, absolutely the most genetically ridiculous man I've ever met at 6'5" and 280lbs of sheer defined muscle and around 5% body fat at the most. We loaded up the leg press with a few plates and he said, "Fifteen reps". I repped out the fifteen without any problem. Then he loads up a few more plates and I say, "How many?" He looked at me quizzically and said, "Fifteen." This time I was pushing myself at the thirteenth, fourteenth and fifteenth and starting to panic because I knew what was coming next: more weight. I said, "Let me guess..." He just laughed and busted out fifteen reps like it was nothing and I realised that day how you get real quads.

Squats are obviously the key here. The king of all exercises has so many benefits beyond just the quads but they are the focal point. Maintain strict form, squat to at least parallel with the floor and complete each rep fully. Leg extensions allow you to achieve peak contraction and isolate the quads, bringing out the separation. Aside from leg extensions, your main movement is a pressing motion, utilised in squats and leg presses. To avoid hitting a plateau, you have to vary the stimulation with using different foot placement (toes pointed outwards targets inner quads, feet together emphasises the outer quads and driving through the heels puts more strain on the hamstrings and brings out the separation between quads and hamstrings. Don't stick to a favourite leg press; many gyms have plate-loaded and cable leg press machines. Use them both; the slightest difference in resistance can make a big difference. Explore repping techniques; try a set with standard cadence, using a machine-like tempo, then use explosive reps, powering up in the positive portion of the rep finally, try slow reps, you will feel all the fibres of the quad rippling and almost tingling. It's a great way to achieve definition.

Hamstrings

When I was doing *Gladiators*, I was humbled very quickly by the athleticism of some of my fellow cast members, most notably, Olympian sprinter and all-round freak of nature Du'aine Ladejo. At 6'0" and about 210lbs, the Barcelona '92 silver medallist could deadlift, squat and bench press powerlifter numbers, and could dunk a basketball. That, boys and girls, is an athlete. I began to analyse him constantly, bugging him with questions. One of the first things I noticed about him was the incredible mass he had in his hamstrings. As someone who has always struggled with adding mass to my sinewy hams, I was green with envy. He told me how in his Olympic days, they would deadlift, but only the positive portion of the lift, dropping the weight at the top because lowering the weight stretched the hamstrings and affected the fast-twitch fibres, which was the primary concern of sprinters. This idea goes completely against the conventional bodybuilding hamstring technique of stretching the hams with stiff-legged deadlifts and good-morning movements, but the results were plain to see; and for the first time I realised the importance of the hamstrings in terms of athletic performance.

Training the Hamstrings

The hamstrings are engaged during squats and deadlifts, particularly when you keep your feet flat and drive through the heels. But for the purpose of directly training the hamstrings, there are two movements: leg curl exercises or stiff legged lifts. Leg curls, either lying or standing, are usually performed with a cable resistance or sometimes plate-loaded. This targets the *biceps femoris* which are sometimes referred to as the 'leg biceps'. This is without doubt the best way to isolate and define the sweep of the hamstring which ties in well with the glute and gives that chiselled athletic look that is desirable in both men and women. The overall mass of the back of the thigh can be attained with stiff-legged deadlifts and good-mornings, an often forgotten move that I think has a myriad of benefits and has made a big comeback in my regimen over the last few months.

With the engagement of the lower back with these moves, I usually train my hamstrings on the same day that I train my back. I have always made better gains by training the quadriceps and hamstrings individually, rather than heaping them all together on 'leg day'. Whatever works for you is fine, but I like to dedicate enough time and energy to both sections of the thighs, as I have such long legs that I have to work hard to make even small gains.

Calves

When it comes to physiques, particularly in men, the calves may be the most controversial muscle of them all. Now I'm speaking as someone who works extremely hard on my calves at least four times per week and still struggles to make even small gains in the lower legs, so I'll choose my words carefully. The calves, much like the forearms, are especially well-conditioned muscles and therefore need a very high stimulation to grow. In other words, you use them all the time so they are already well prepared for anything so it's hard to get them to change. Their growth and response to training is also extremely dependent on your genetics (cue the scoffs from all the guys out there with great calves who work them once or twice a week!).

I know it sounds like a cop-out but it's true. Perhaps this also ties in with the fact that they are also one of the most neglected muscles when it comes to training; because some people achieve great calves almost effortlessly, it further discourages the people at the other end of the spectrum as they start to think, "What's the point, they're not going to grow anyway?" But this is the wrong approach...

Training the Calves

If, like me, you're never going to have calves that look like your knee swallowed a grapefruit it doesn't mean you shouldn't be training them with as much intensity as everything else. In fact, you should be training them more frequently and prioritising them, training them at the beginning when you're fresh. There is really only one exercise, the calf raise, but there are many variations such as one-legged, machine, seated and others and I suggest you apply them all, using multiple intensity techniques and principles to shock them. Remember, they are already very strong and conditioned, so they need to be subjected to something that really throws them off kilter. In my experience, drop sets seems to be the best way to do this. Frank Zane, widely regarded as one of the most aesthetic physiques of all time, also professed this method. It's important to take the calf through the full range of motion; stretching at the bottom and lifting them as high as you can go on your toes to get that full contraction. Partial reps are OK in limited numbers, but if you don't take the gastrocnemius through the full range, a lot of the work is going to be taken on by the soleus muscles on either side of the shin and Achilles tendon. I'm appreciative of the performance benefits of training the calves; I have to be on the balls of my feet and able to have good footwork. As I write this, I'm recovering from a torn PCL in my knee and part of my rehab is to build more strength in the accompanying muscles of the lower leg like the *tibialis anterior, peroneus* and *extensor*. I highly recommend that you do reverse calf raises (place your heels on the platform and raise your toes from the floor up) because remember, as the rest of your major muscles grow, your smaller muscles have to cope with a higher weight and if there is too much of a difference, the joint suffers. I'm speaking from experience.

Biceps

Whether we like to admit it or not, the bicep will forever be the poster boy of muscle development. The bicep pose is hit more frequently than duck face during a selfie, and the last time I checked, when someone says, 'Show me your muscles,' people aren't dropping their trousers and flexing their quads in the bar, although if you ever do that and I'm in that bar, I will pay for all your drinks all night!

If you're reading this book, the chances are you appreciate a full, lean bicep and want to achieve the same look for yourself. And yes, while I may have commented on the fact that women appreciate less common areas of the physique, the fact still remains that if they're into athletic-bodied men, one of the first things they're going to want is a decent gun to hang on to. Speaking of women, ladies all over the world have embraced the fact that a lean, athletic arm is sexy on a female physique too, especially considering that women's arms are actually on full display more often than men's when you take into account all the strappy dresses (unfortunately, this book will not reduce the time it takes for them to get ready, if it did I'd be a billionaire).

Training the Biceps

Although you may want big bulging bis, relatively speaking they are a small muscle in the body, and there is really one move (the bicep curl with a myriad of variations) that works them. This is why the most common mistake I see from guys who want to improve their biceps is a lack of volume and/or intensity. Your biceps are stimulated when you train your back, and even when you're performing regular day-to-day tasks like putting things on shelves etc. So they're actually quite well-conditioned, which means they need to be challenged to really respond. This means using a challenging weight, and training with enough volume (sets/reps) and using different training principles to shock the biceps. Some people use too much weight, doing set after set of cheat curls. Their back is probably getting a great workout, but the bis, not so much. Conversely, many trainers are all about the isolation, doing preacher curls, isolation curls, single arm cable curls and using strict form. While the bicep may improve in terms of definition, it's going to lack that thickness and fullness that completes the arm. Treat the bicep like any other muscle group; respect the compound lift (heavy barbell curls) and then sculpt with isolation moves. Remember to use heavy hammer curls to target the forearm and the *brachialis*, which sits between the bicep and tricep and achieves that thick, chiselled arm that you saw wielding a machine gun one-handed in *Predator* or *Rambo*. Sometimes you have to work through 'the pump' with biceps. I realised that my arms were stuck in a rut because I was not doing enough sets, and it was mainly because I would have this phenomenal pump after about twelve sets, so instinctively I would wind down, when in fact I had to power through and go for sixteen or more working sets. If your forearms are doing too much of the work it's going to harm your bicep development, so focus on relaxing the wrist and mentally focusing on the engagement of the bicep. Finally, remember that the bicep is also responsible for rotating the wrist, so incorporate twisting motions with your dumbbell curl (Zottman curls are a great option) and focus on the full range of motion and peak contraction.

Triceps

I don't want to patronise you, but I want to make the following statement to emphasise a point that should always be on your mind when you're thinking about your arms: *three is more than two.* The bicep has two heads, the tricep has three. So in basic terms, 3/5 of your upper arm is tricep and 2/5 is bicep. Are you respecting your triceps enough?

Because of my genetics, I was always naturally pretty lean, which meant that I could see my tricep development very quickly, which was fortunate because it encouraged me to always relish my tricep training. Watching wrestling as a kid, I always wanted that pumped, chiselled look in the upper arm that guys like The Rock had when they were wearing a sleeveless shirt, most of which comes from great triceps development (Rock has always had great upper arms for such a tall guy). You can't walk around flexing your biceps 24/7, so you better have equally impressive tris if you're going to have arms that command attention.

Training the Triceps

I look at tricep training the same way I look at shoulder training; there are so many options to build and sculpt the tris that with a little experience it should become easy and you should look forward to triceps days. Triceps are engaged when you do any kind of pushing or pressing movement e.g. bench press, so there are pressing movements you can do that target the tris like close-grip bench press, but the extension of the arm is also the primary responsibility of the tricep and it is with this movement that you will achieve real growth and shape. You should be looking to achieve a horseshoe-like appearance at the back of the arm, indicating equal development of all three heads of the tricep. There is such a huge variety that you should easily be able to challenge the tris differently every time. The outer head (the one you see from the side) is mostly engaged by pressing movements. The upper head (the top of the horseshoe) comes from getting a full contraction in extension movements like rope press down. The inner head seems to respond better for me with dumbbell movements like overhead dumbbell extension or kick backs. Explore for yourself which movements hit the areas best for you from the *Build Your Workout Reference Table* and remember that for almost every tricep exercise, you can change it up by doing the same exercise with a different type of resistance. For example, swap dumbbells for cables, cables for a barbell and try dips on TRX straps or rings. One of my favourites is to perform bodyweight tricep extensions on gymnastics rings instead of a straight bar. The first time I tried it I could only manage about five reps, and that was after ten years of training!

Forearms

A rival of calves in the stubbornness department, forearms work so much in day-to-day life that it takes specific targeted effort to make them adapt. In addition, they share the other common characteristic of their cousins south of the border, which is that genetics play a big part; there are some guys who have never performed a specific forearm exercise in their life and have monstrous, defined forearms while many of us toil away with a host of exercises to make even minimal improvements. But hey, if being in shape was easy, everybody would be doing it. So whether it comes easily or not, training your forearms is a must if you want complete arms from top to bottom, because it means nothing if what you've got up top isn't at least complemented by what's down below.

Training the Forearms

There are a lot of smaller muscles that make up the forearms but let's keep it simple; the main focus is the flexors, on the underside of the forearm that pull the hand toward the bicep and the extensors on the outer side of the forearm that lift the back of the hand upwards. Both are worked during most upper body lifts but to target them specifically the best exercise is the wrist curl (flexor) and reverse wrist curl (extensor) which can be performed with a barbell, dumbbell or cables. Adding hammer curls and reverse grip curls to your biceps workout will challenge the forearms and one of my personal favourites is isometric plate holds; take two 10lb Olympic plates and put them together and hold them with one hand by your side for as long as possible. It will burn your forearms and improve your grip strength, and you can progress to more weight or additional plates to challenge the forearms in different ways as your strength improves.

Trapezius (Traps)

Ever since a snorting, snarling, 290lb phenomenon called Bill Goldberg emerged as one of the biggest stars in pro wrestling during the 1990s I've understood and respected what a pair of traps can do for your look. First and foremost, proportion is fundamentally important to a good physique so if you're planning on building your chest, shoulders and upper arms, you better get your traps up to scratch or you'll always look like a wannabe. I know this from first-hand experience; when I look back at 21-year-old me from *Gladiators* I cringe at how pencil-necked I was. People would always say to me, "Wow, you're much bigger than you look on TV," and I realised that one of the main reasons for this was that at least half of my individual screen time was focused on my face, so I looked like an average guy from the neck up which didn't sit well with me. I prioritised my traps and now I'm happy to say that they are in proportion with my chest and shoulders, and I don't feel like an average guy any more.

Traps imply power; a thick neck tells people you're serious and not just going through the motions. We've all seen that one guy, who is wearing an extra-medium shirt, has a big chest and biceps but still looks...goofy. Chances are he's never done a shrug in his life, apart from when you asked him when the last time he trained traps was.

Training the Traps

The trapezius' main job is to lift the shoulders, so naturally your weapon of choice is shrugs. The key things to remember with shrugs are to use a heavy weight (it's the only way they will respond) and to take the shrug through the full range of motion. If you don't stretch at the bottom and lift all the way to your ears, you won't get that smooth sweep down the neck that you want with good traps. My personal favourite way to shrug is with heavy dumbbells, but you can use a barbell, a smith machine or even cables, all of which offer a slightly different type of resistance which will add muscularity and shape. Sometimes I even use the standing calf raise machine, placing the pads on my shoulders and shrugging that way, which I find hits the back of my neck and traps more which is obviously beneficial to protecting myself in wrestling. Much like calves, forearms and other areas that don't get the spotlight, one of the common mistakes I see is people simply don't give their traps enough volume; not enough sets, not enough reps, not enough weight. Dedicate some time to them and watch them respond rapidly.

Abs and Core

Superstar Spotlight – Rob Strauss aka Robbie E

TV Ready Midsection by ROBBIE E

The key is to be born an absolutely drop dead SEXY specimen of perfect genetics like I am! Then you can skip leg days, cardio and eat whatever you want!

I wish that were true! The most important thing is obviously a healthy balanced diet. Try to avoid sugar as much as possible. Any time you ingest something that tastes "sweet", your brain tells your body to release insulin! Obvious things like white bread and beer are a big ENEMY of fat-burning, even a big bowl of rice, and an extended period without food is no good. Insulin release automatically shuts down your fat-burning capacity and keeps it in low gear for quite a while, while actually promoting fat storage. Stay AWAY from sweet stuff, eat vegetables and lean meats, keep lifting weights but throw in some High Intensity Interval Training (HIIT) to your cardio routine! Try 8-10 sets of 30-second sprints with 60-90 seconds of rest in between. Do all that, and with a little luck you MAY someday look as AMAZING as I do!

Robbie E ABDOMINAL Workout (After Sprints)
*Perform Each Exercise for 30 seconds each with no break in between exercises

(Perform the entire circuit 3 times – 3 days/week)
1. Bicycle Twists
2. Mountain Climbers
3. Crush/Reverse Crunch (More Advanced)
4. Planks/One Arm Planks (More Advanced)

Rob Strauss aka Robbie E, TNA Impact Wrestling Star, Star of The Amazing Race on CBS. Robbie offers personalised training and diet plans – get one by emailing him at RobbieEFitness@gmail.com Twitter.com/robbieeimpact Instagram.com/robbieeimpact Official Website – robbie-e.com Facebook – Subscribe and Friend Request http:// www.facebook.com/robbie.eimpact.1

Because you are reading this, I assume you're either already into fitness and nutrition or you are looking to improve your body and want some helpful information. Either way, because you are reading this I can be pretty sure that a great midsection is high on your body wish list. Whether you want a ripped, washboard six-pack or simply a lean, flat stomach you are not alone; it's one of the first things I'm asked about by most people who ask advice. It should come as no surprise that because of the strong desire for a great core in so many people that there is such a huge amount of information and opinion out there – it is easily the most contested area of the body in terms of advice and opinion. One thing is for certain, however; great abs remain one of the most sought-after holy grails of fitness.

Training the Abs and Core

There are always hundreds of abs routines available every month in fitness magazines, as well as "abs in one move" promises and all kinds of other sure-fire formulas. On the other hand, a lot of old-school guys will say something to the effect of, "Your abs get worked when you lift weights, it's just your body fat that will bring them out or not." As with most things, the reality lies somewhere in the middle; yes, if you do a lot of standing moves and use free weights, your *rectus abdominus* will have to work to aid you and support you, but that's not going to build and sculpt the abs to get the desired look. However, don't toil away with hundreds of endless crunches, it's a waste of time. My key points to keeping your core in line:

- *Treat the abdominals like every other muscle.* They need resistance, moves that focus on the upper, lower and middle and they need to be taken through the full range of motion. I see a lot of guys' routines that include a nominal amount of crunches or something similar tacked on to the end of a workout. Would you treat your biceps that way? No. So don't treat your abs that way. Do a defined number of exercises, sets and reps and apply the same principles to abs that you apply to all other muscles.

- *Train your core, not your abs.* For a long time, a lot of people (myself included) were only concerned with the abs and, even worse, were predominantly concerned with the visual aspect, not understanding how vital a strong core is to your performance in so many things. Thankfully people are more aware now but it bears repeating that whether you're an athlete or just looking to improve your physique from an aesthetic standpoint, start looking at your core as the area to train, not 'abs'. Good abs mean nothing if they're not accompanied by good obliques and intercostals, and supported by a strong transverse abdominus (the sheet of muscle that lies behind your rectus abdominus and is responsible for holding your stomach in).

- *Train your core year-round, not just in the summer time.* Just because you're not planning to be shirtless in the winter, or if you decide to focus on adding mass in the winter like many do, don't neglect your midsection. It will hinder your progress in other areas, and when the spring rolls around, if your core is neglected it will take you all that time to get it back, which means by the time your midsection is up to scratch, the summer is over and your shirt is back on.

My favourite way to train my core is in a circuit: The abs and core muscles are engaged so much in my day-to-day activities like lifting weights, wrestling etc that to really get them to respond I have to hit them hard and keep the rest period to a minimum, so circuits seem to work best for me. I try to set up about four or five exercises, comprising one exercise for obliques, one exercise that targets upper, middle and lower abs respectively and one core strength exercise to strengthen the transverse abdominus and bring out overall definition and separation in my midsection. Here's an example: 1) Ab Wheel Roll Out x 15 reps 2) Standing Twists x 50 (25 each side) 3) Jackknife sit ups x 15 reps 4) Reverse crunch x 15 reps 5) Plank for 1 minute. Complete each exercise consecutively, perform entire circuit five times, resting one or two minutes between each circuit or as long as you need, but challenge yourself.

Remember to keep it varied; the core needs to be challenged in new ways all the time to stay responsive. To be able to 'see' your abs you need low body fat, typically under 10%. But that is more dependent on cardio and diet which we'll cover separately.

Cardio

As you forge ahead in your pursuit for your superstar body, you will hopefully understand that the best bodies come from a synergy of effective training, diet and lifestyle, hence the mantra *Train Eat Live*. But each one of those three areas contains a larger number of elements within them that also need to act harmoniously to be most effective. Within The *Train* section, obviously the bulk of the content focuses on weight training, because there are a lot more details to cover.

But now it's time to discuss the other key area of training that is vital to not only a great physique, but to your overall health and wellbeing. An area that for some inspires great excitement and for others strikes fear in their soon-to-be pumping heart. I'm of course referring to cardio.

The Steady-State Debate

There is a long-standing belief that doing steady-state 'easy' cardio, like walking on a treadmill or doing the elliptical trainer for long periods of time at low intensity, is better for burning fat. You will even see this ideal written on many cardio machines in commercial gyms; you know, the little chart that says that 65% of maximum heart rate (MRH) is the 'fat burning zone' and 85% of MRH is the 'cardio zone'.

This is a myth. Forget this idea forever.

Okay, I'm not suggesting that you can never do steady-state cardio. I myself will regularly watch Netflix or do some wrestling video study whilst walking on a treadmill or doing the elliptical trainer, but I'm not under any illusion that I'm going to be shredded by doing that. If it were that simple, wouldn't you see more people with superstar bodies? If you want to have an extraordinary physique, you need to do things most people aren't willing to do. But that's not the only reason to avoid doing too much steady-state cardio. Here are some more:

1. It's catabolic, which means muscle-wasting. Yes, you read that correctly, *it takes away your hard-earned muscle!*

2. It releases cortisol. I'm not going to bore you with a ton of scientific babble about the stress hormone cortisol, but just know this; it's bad. So bad in fact that it is one of the arch enemies of a good physique, because cortisol is catabolic AND causes fatty deposits in the most prone area (stomach for men, thighs and butt for women). Add to that water retention and wave goodbye to the superstar body in your mind's eye.

Steady-state cardio is OK now and then. It's good for your heart because you can get it up to a good heart rate for a sustained period of time which is good for the circulation. I also find that it allows me to generate some overall heat in my body and gives me a little more fluidity and elasticity in my muscles and joints which is why I do it a couple of times per week. But make no mistake, I do it to avoid sitting on the couch, not for an effective workout. For real results, in both performance and physique, you need to challenge yourself just like you do in the weight room.

Intensity = Intensity

Superstar Spotlight: David McIntosh

Boys, girls and extremely talented gentlemen, there are many effective ways to keep the body fat low so that the solid vascular muscle you've spent ages working on in the gym gets a chance to shine right on through. I'm gonna give you a couple of real sweet tips to make that dream body come to life.

One means of getting seriously shredded is through your diet, of course. I would never say go carb free but 100% be carb careful. Limit yourself to one carb meal a day, preferably earlier on in the day so it gives you a good steady release of power throughout and you're still able to smash the big boy weights no matter what time. Juicing is also a key factor: not fruit juice or any whack ass juice from the grocery store. I'm talking about daily selecting an array of fresh vegetables, preferably organic, and juicing them yourself. This will help shed your body of waste products which can be anywhere up to 11lbs!

The more painful way to becoming a shredded God of old is upping your intensity when training. My sessions are no longer than an hour, but it ain't no walk in the park. I enter a realm of pain, blood, sweat and pumps that blow your eyeballs out! I tend to mix a heavy weighted exercise with an own body weight exercise. For instance, I would superset heavy squats 5-10 reps with 30 seconds of tuck jumps immediately after. If I was training back I would do heavy seated rows followed by jumping straight on to the pull-up bar, same kind of rep range. This kind of training will keep your heart rate pumping at optimum levels and shed that fat like a son of a god damn wasp!

Magnus: thanks for letting me hit your readers with some bad boy tips and also allowing me to feature in this electric fitness bible.

David McIntosh, former Royal Marines Commando, actor, television personality including Gladiators and Celebrity Big Brother, fitness model including Muscle and Fitness cover model.
Website: www.kingdavidmcintosh.com
Twitter: @devildawg85
Instagram: @king_david85

While my old pal Tosh might be talking about his weight training rather than cardio specifically, it's a perfect example of something you need to get in your head if you want a body that stands out (and I think we can all agree that David's physique, like his writing style, raises a few eyebrows). **Ramping up the intensity for even one hour in the gym is so much more effective than plodding away for endless hours doing something easy.**

Remember how I talked about *maximising your minutes?* This applies especially well to cardio. Think about it this way: If you want to look like a professional athlete, when was the last time you saw a bunch of professional athletes on row after row of elliptical trainers in the gym? Challenge yourself, make yourself breathe heavily, push yourself to the point where you are really sucking that precious oxygen in. You can get a greater overall benefit from ten minutes of this than an hour plodding away on a machine watching *ESPN*.

Why? For me, there are two primary reasons. The first is that much like with your weight training, you have to shock the body into adapting. To shed unwanted body fat and increase definition in the key area, you need to shock the body into thinking, "Oh my God, I can't cope with this in my current state, I need to adapt!" The second reason ties in with the first, which is that lots of credible research has shown that after performing high-intensity cardio, your *Basal Metabolic Rate (BMR)* stays elevated for longer afterwards. In a nutshell, your BMR is the amount of calories you burn while doing nothing. So as long as you're consuming enough protein to maintain your muscle mass, a higher BMR will lead to more fat being melted away.

The solution for optimum physique results: HIIT

High Intensity Interval Training, or HIIT, is a way to effectively and practically utilise the aforementioned facts and advice. It's tough to push yourself to the absolute limit for a long period of time, day after day, without overtraining or hitting a wall and slowing your overall progress in the long term. By using HIIT, you will perform bursts of activity at the highest possible intensity and superset it with slower steady periods. This allows you to get the benefits of pushing yourself, but subject your body to it for a longer period so you can elicit an adaptation from your body.

Have you looked at top level sprinters lately? I think we can all agree that those guys look good. So it should carry some weight that HIIT is derived from sprint training concepts that have been used for decades, most notably the *Peter Coe regimen* that was used to train the legendary British athlete Sebastian Coe. Other well-known regimens include the *Tabata, Gibala* and *Timmons Regimens.*

HIIT can be utilised in an infinite amount of ways, but some examples include:

Sprints: 100m (or any distance) sprints

x 10 with 30 seconds rest in between.

High knees for 20 seconds, walk for 10 seconds, repeat 10 times.

Treadmill: My personal favourite is to set the treadmill to a high incline, then run for 90 seconds, walk for 1 minute. Obviously there are endless variations to this technique.

My get-lean circuit: Burpees x10, 40lb Medicine Ball Slam x 10, Jump Rope x 100. Rest 1 minute. Repeat 5 times.

So as you can see, traditional cardio methods as well as bodyweight resistance and even weighted resistance moves can be utilised. The key is to work at a very high anaerobic intensity for a short period of time then take short rests or periods of lower intensity. Your heart rate will go through the roof and you will sweat! If you typically try to stay to a minimum of 2:1 ratio of work to rest you are on the right track. To challenge yourself you can up the ratio to 3:1 or even more.

Benefits of HIIT include:

3. Increased BMR – Many credible studies from both coaches and physiologists have concluded that HIIT can increase resting metabolism for as long as 24 hours after your HIIT workout. In basic terms, your furnace is burning all day. So put the work in for 30 minutes of HIIT, then you'll be burning fat while you're tweeting, watching *Modern Family*, stalking your ex on Facebook or whatever else you're doing when you're not reading this book or training.

4. Improved insulin sensitivity – I'm not an expert on this by any means, but insulin is hugely important to your health as well as your physique. In layman's terms, insulin sensitivity is good, insulin resistance is bad. HIIT has been shown to reduce insulin resistance, which causes fat gain, internal bloating and high blood sugar which can lead to diabetes.

5. Improved muscle oxidative capacity – in other words, you will be good for **show** and for go.

I've visited hundreds of fitness websites and publications, but in my opinion I have found the most compelling reading on HIIT, Sprint Training and other tremendous cardio tips at www.simplyshredded.com.

Part 2

EAT

Introduction

Tell me what you eat, and I will tell you who you are. – Jean Antheime Brillat-Savarin

Welcome to the biggest information minefield in the world today. Ever since we as humans evolved beyond eating merely for survival, there has been a fork in the road for human exploration of food; those who seek to discover how to make it taste as good as possible, and those who investigate what effect that food has on our bodies. I tip my hat to both.

Before we get into this section, I want to take a moment to reflect on the fact that if you're reading this book, the chances are you're one of the people in the world fortunate enough to enjoy a choice of when and what you eat. As we ponder what food to buy, how to prepare it and cook it, always be aware that there are many in the world not as fortunate. My knowledge and appreciation of food and cooking is a direct result of being raised by good parents with a healthy approach to food and being fortunate enough to afford it. Many kids are not afforded that same opportunity. If this is something that grabs you, visit www.nokidhungry.org (US) or www.savethechildren.org.uk (UK and Worldwide) and help however you can.

As I alluded to at the beginning of this introduction, diet and nutrition at every level is a minefield of information (and misinformation). The main reason for this? Like so many other hot-button topics in the world, *follow the money...*

You see, food is one of those things that people will always need to buy, and the market is incredibly competitive. So as health and wellness starts to become a larger part of public consciousness, 'facts' and 'guidelines' are interpreted to fit the agenda of the companies trying to sell you their products. Sometimes, these facts are completely created by the companies themselves. Look, I love a bowl of cereal as much as the next guy (I'm still a big kid at heart) but when cereal commercials try and tell parents that their bowl of sugar is good for growing kids because it has some calcium in it, or the middle-aged guy in the commercial is going to escape heart disease by eating a bowl, I'm throwing the flag on that play.

What you eat is equally important as what you do in the gym. That doesn't mean that you have to miserably chow your way through plain chicken breast and spinach every day. It means you have to develop a fundamental understanding of a few key things when it comes to nutrition, and it would serve you well to know how to cook. One of my best friends, Tom, moved to Florida from the UK around the same time as me, is the same age, height, weight and has similar proportions. We're very similar in a lot of ways, but our approach to eating is drastically different: mainly because the guy doesn't know a frying pan from a bed pan! He can't cook! Subsequently, he subjects himself to the most plain, unappetising meals known to man and then eventually cracks and gorges on all the junk he can get his hands on. Every time he comes to my place, I'll make us something to eat and he'll remark on how good it is. Every time I go to his place, he offers to make me something to eat, and I say, "Erm, how about we go out to eat?"

The way you approach your food intake should be exactly the same way you approach your workouts; some things will work for you, some won't. This is something that a lot of people get stuck on with food: *every single person reacts differently to what they eat just as they do to exercise.* There are no set rules you absolutely have to follow. What you eat is not just about the nutrients within that food, but also about your body's hormonal response to the food. This may be the biggest piece of information many people don't know about. I'll explain some more on this as we move forward.

I promised that this book wouldn't overload you with information, simply give you the necessary tools you need to build the body you want and put you in control of it. Trust me, it really is a great feeling to know that you have complete control over your body, to be able to say, "I can drop ten pounds in two weeks if I need to simply by making a few small adjustments to my diet." I should know, I just did that. I tore my PCL in my right knee, so while I was rehabbing it I decided to drop a little weight to take some pressure off and went from 250lbs to 240. This isn't bragging; in fact, there's nothing to brag about, I don't see 'losing weight' as an accomplishment. Changing your body is an accomplishment;and besides, ten pounds as a percentage of 254 per cent. But I'm illustrating a point that once you know how your body reacts to not only what you subject it to in the gym or wherever you exercise, but what you feed it too, you can make significant changes.

The EAT Principles

A crust eaten in peace is better than a banquet partaken in anxiety – Aesop

I could have written individual sections on each of the following but I decided that you need the essential information and it needs to be easily digested, so I put what I believe to be the most important need-to-know points into this section as principles that I believe will help you get control of your body by what you put into it.

- **Forget calories** – Using calories as any significant way to justify what you're eating is going to get you nowhere. Measuring calories is outdated and a waste of time. Still not sold? I'll elaborate; the calorie was first defined by Nicolas Clement in 1824. Yes, you read that right, *1824*, when people were dying of smallpox and Stonewall Jackson was being born. It was first defined as a unit of heat, but in food context it is a unit of energy. There are in fact two different types of calorie; one is used in chemistry, the dietary calorie is actually called a large calorie. Even more confusing is the fact that in nutrition contexts, a Kilojoule is the recognised unit of food energy, and calories despite being in common use to this day are *not even officially recognised as a unit of food energy*. Unfortunately, somewhere along the way, somebody made the connection between calories and food and used it to suggest approximate amounts of calories required in basic nutritional requirements for survival. The information was taken completely out of context over time and now our society worships this almighty number of calories like it's an exact science.

Sure, probably the most basic approach to weight loss (or gain) is calorie deficit (or surplus) which just means if you want to lose weight, the amount of calories you burn has to exceed the amount you eat or vice versa if you wish to gain weight. But in *10 To Remember* I said worship the mirror, not the scales. We're not trying to be concerned with just how much we physically weigh, we're trying to change our physiques; weight change is a byproduct. So we have to look beyond this outdated, irrelevant information.

- **Quality protein is the key** – Remember that the fundamental approach is to think like a sculptor; to add lean mass and then chisel down around it. Protein provides amino acids, which are the building materials you need. Not to get into too much jargon here but to support and facilitate muscle growth your body needs to be in a state of *positive nitrogen balance* also known as *nitrogen retention*. Basically, protein is the only macro nutrient that contains nitrogen; more nitrogen needs to be retained than expelled for muscle growth. The way you do this is by a) stimulating as many muscle fibres as possible without causing muscle breakdown and b) consuming enough protein to provide your muscle fibres with the amino acids they need to achieve positive nitrogen balance. Remember, if you're subjecting your body to daily workouts, your protein requirements are significantly higher than any "Recommended Daily Allowance" (I hate that term). Typically, the most agreed ratio for protein consumption is one gram for every pound of body weight. I like to treat this as a strict minimum, and if I can, go for about 1.5 grams.

You also need to understand that not all proteins are created equal; each protein source has a Biological Value (BV) which in basic terms means the amount of the protein that can be used by the body. The *Typical Value* refers to it as a percentage, which in my opinion is the easier way to display BV of proteins. As an example, here are the big hitters: whey protein 96%, eggs 94%, cow's milk 90%. As a way to emphasise why it's important to know this, chicken has a BV of 79%, beef 74% and most common fish sources are around 76%. For vegetarians BV has to be a concern: while whole soybean protein has a high BV of 96%, soybean curd (tofu) is only 64%. This is the main reason I try to exceed the minimum of one gram per pound of bodyweight; because while some of my protein intake is from whey protein and eggs, some is from less valuable sources, so I know some of the protein is not being used.

- **Eat real food** – A common mistake many people make is to get too many of their target grams of protein from bars or shakes. I should know; I was guilty of this for a long time, and it was why I was so frustrated with my lack of density and fullness, especially if I tried to lean out for a big match, photo shoot or just for the beach.

  It's important to get as many of your macronutrients as possible from whole food sources. It will result in a better quality look due to better muscle composition, not to mention the fact that you will get all the extra micronutrients, vitamins and minerals from whole food sources that you won't get from shakes and bars. While we're on the subject, I try to avoid protein bars for the most part; they're mainly comprised of dehydrated protein and binding agents that are hard to digest. For the money, you're not getting quality, muscle-building food. If I'm travelling, and a protein bar is the best option at an airport for example, I make sure to drink plenty of water with the bar. While there are some great quality protein powders available today, I still try and limit my shakes to two per day; usually after a workout and before bed. It's tempting to think that you can just get half of your daily protein requirements from shakes and continue to eat three meals a day like the rest of society. Unfortunately, the rest of society don't have superstar bodies. If you want one, you're going to have to be different. Eat good quality protein, carb and fat sources and chew it properly; chewing exposes the food to saliva which contains digestive enzymes including lingual lipase, an enzyme that helps break down fat.

- **Eat more fat** – For so many years, the word 'fat'
  when it comes to nutrition has been the edible
  Antichrist. Unfortunately our English language
  is mostly to blame. Bear with me on this, as it's
  a theory I've formulated over time and I really
  think it holds weight (no pun intended)...Because
  we use the word 'fat' to describe people who
  are overweight or, more specifically, people with
  excess adipose tissue (body fat), the word 'fat'
  when describing the key macronutrient found in
  foods has automatically been linked to making
  you 'fat' in the physical way. Make sense? I truly
  believe that if we had simply used a different
  word to describe dietary fat, we would have had
  way less problems, more understanding and
  more appreciation of this vital and valuable
  nutrient. Please get rid of the over-simplified
  notion that eating fat makes you fat.

  Fat is fantastic.

  Fat is necessary for so many vital functions
  of the body; it allows you to absorb certain
  nutrients, most notably vitamins A, D, E and K.
  Fat is needed to maintain a steady core body
  temperature and fat is a valuable source of
  energy, which leads me to one of the ways we
  have been so misled for so long: I remember
  back when I was in high school learning about
  the food groups and they would give you a basic
  rundown of Carbohydrates, Fats and Protein.
  I always remember carbohydrates being the
  most associated with 'energy', while fat had
  energy listed as one of its purposes but the
  implication was that it was slow energy and
  you needed carbohydrate for real energy. This

is a fundamentally wrong consensus. Much in the same way that the word 'fat' has too many connotations, the word 'energy' is also misrepresented. Up until recently, I would always start my day with some protein and carbohydrate, under the assumption that it would provide me with some energy throughout the day. After becoming an ambassador for Bulletproof, and learning from biohacker and mad genius Dave Asprey, I realised that by starting my day with protein and good fats, I am full of energy, my mind is switched on and not foggy and I don't feel bloated. I'm still consuming enough to maintain my size and fuel my workouts. But I'm leaner without working any harder. And it's all thanks to eating more fat and less carbohydrates.

I should point out that saying 'eat more fat' is over-simplistic. Obviously you have to limit your carbohydrate intake or you'll over-eat and gain unwanted weight. Also, there are fats that are incredibly valuable and have a myriad of benefits, and there are some which are just plain bad for you and contribute to obesity, bad cholesterol, decreased liver function and all the nasty stuff that can come as a result of those issues. One thing we have to do is focus on Essential Fatty Acids (EFAs) which are important for the body to function and have to be obtained from food as they can't be produced by the body. Eating foods rich in Omega 3, 6 and 9 fatty acids is the best way to go, but there are also some benefits to consuming some natural saturated animal fat, most notably hormonal. Testosterone production is optimised by consuming monounsaturated fats and even saturated fats like those found in red meat and egg yolks. We'll cover this in more detail in the EAT Food Table and sample meal plans, but for now start getting on board with the idea that eating the right fat is not only delicious but vital for your performance and physique goals.

- **Understand carbohydrates and insulin** – Ah, the great carb debate! What kind of carbs, when to eat them, how much, whether to eat them at all... the arguments rage on. But as is the case with most things, you will have to see what works for you, but understanding them in a little more depth will help. I want to explain how carbs affect body fat so much; enter insulin.

  OK, I promised I wouldn't bog you down with too much science, so I'll try to use broad strokes but this is important. Insulin is a hormone produced in the pancreas that regulates metabolism. Insulin does several things but one of them is it causes fat to be stored rather than used for energy: not good. It also inhibits growth hormone production, and seeing as growth hormone is just about the best thing in the body (cell replenishment, muscle mass, reduced body fat and anti-aging) this is really not good. Now this may sound a little counter-intuitive but the state we want to achieve if we want to be in great shape is *insulin sensitivity*. What we want to avoid is *insulin resistance*.

  Insulin resistance is when cells fail to respond to the normal actions of insulin and the result is high blood sugar AND the pancreas produces even more insulin. The main risk of this is of course Type 2 diabetes. But even in smaller amounts, insulin resistance will lead to a number of symptoms, most notably intestinal bloating, weight gain from high fat storage and increased hunger, making a vicious cycle ready to destroy your visions of a Greek god physique.

There are many contributing factors to insulin resistance but we're going to focus on elevated blood glucose levels from *excessive regular carbohydrate intake*. I used italics there so that you get the point that eating carbs ever is not going to be a problem, but regularly over-filling your body with carbs it doesn't need is going to be a problem. I've used this analogy before when advising people: If you take a funnel and pour oil into it, it will flow through. There may be some residue left over, but it will eventually go through. If you add flour to that oil, it will get clogged and some will be left behind. Think of your body as the funnel. But we do need carbs sometimes to fuel us though intense workouts and replenish muscle glycogen, ensuring that desired 'full' look in the muscle belly. My personal favourite technique to find the happy medium of getting the carbs you need to fuel your workouts, keep fullness in your muscles without gaining body fat is *carb cycling* which I will cover in more detail.

- **Control your sugar** – Directly related to the last point, sugar is the fastest way to raise blood sugar levels and cause the problems associated with excess insulin release. Sugar is what is known as an 'empty calorie', it has no essential nutrients but a huge amount of energy, which, unused, can be a fast track to unwanted body fat and a stronger reliance on sugar from the constant rise and dip in blood sugar levels, often referred to as the 'blood sugar rollercoaster'.

I'm not suggesting you cut sugar completely; in fact, a small amount after a workout can sometimes be both necessary and effective as it helps transport the protein you should be taking in and any other nutrients more quickly.

Sugar is found in so many things that it's important to understand when you're eating sugar, not just when you're eating foods with added sugar. For example, fruit and dairy both contain natural sugars in fructose and lactose respectively. While it's definitely preferable over refined sugar (natural sugars help transport the nutrients found in those food sources) you still need to avoid excess consumption. Refined sugars are the real villain here; regular white sugar is refined from sugar cane or sugar beets and high fructose corn syrup is the sugar of choice for a lot of food companies that add sugar to things like soda and sweet products. I should also point out that the 'diet' or 'low fat' options on shelves is often full of this stuff which in all likelihood will make you more fat and more miserable in the long run than just eating some good natural fat. In recent years there has been a rise in popularity of 'organic' and 'raw' sugar. Many people assume this means it has not been processed but this is not true. In the US, the FDA labels raw sugar as unfit for direct consumption due to impurities, so they're still refined and processed before sale. So the 'natural', 'organic' and 'raw' sugars you pay more money for are actually referring to their farming methods used to grow the beets or cane, grown without pesticides or herbicides and refined in a way that doesn't remove all the natural molasses content, unlike white sugar. Either way, always check labels for sugar; you will be amazed at some of the amounts in foods you never even associated with sugar.

- **Change it up** – Like I alluded to earlier, you have to approach your diet the same way you approach your workouts; get a solid grip of the fundamentals of good nutrition, then adjust the additional intake to suit your current needs. Just like somebody who mindlessly goes through the motions of the same workout day in and day out, you cannot expect to see significant improvement in muscle mass, body fat reduction, greater energy levels or even general wellbeing if you're mindlessly eating the same stuff all the time. This is another common sticking point I see in a lot of people. If you eat eggs or egg whites in the morning, then chicken and vegetables three times a day, accompanied by two or three protein shakes, I tip my hat to you for your dedication, but you're missing out on all kinds of micronutrients that come from different varieties within food groups. Last night, before I wrote this section, I went to the supermarket to get something for dinner (I try to buy fruit and vegetables fresh almost daily) and I decided I felt like red cabbage, even though I had never cooked it. I just looked up a recipe online on how to sauté it with red onions, olive oil and apple cider vinegar, and it was delicious! I could have just bought broccoli or spinach like I often do, but I decided I would benefit from eating some red vegetables. This is just an example of what I'm suggesting; go for different types of meat, different cuts, try all the different vegetables that are out there, they all provide slightly different nutrients. Cook things in different ways, all it takes is a few minutes online (I usually just Google it but I most frequently find myself using a recipe on www.foodnetwork. com).

- **Stay hydrated** – It should be common sense to understand the need to drink plenty of water, especially when undertaking a lot of physical output. Your performance both mentally and physically will suffer if your brain, organs and muscles are not adequately hydrated.

  One commonly overlooked issue with achieving great definition is water retention. Often, subcutaneous (under the skin) water is mistaken for body fat because it causes a similar look; an undesirable one, unless you want to look like an unmade bed.

  There are several causes for water retention; some are hormonal, some are environmental. But the best way to ensure that you don't retain water is by drinking plenty of unadulterated water. Your body is very smart and very adaptive; just like with essential fats, if the body is

deprived of water it will hold on to the water
it has in order to stay cool and the first place
it goes is under the skin. Drink more, lose the
wobbly bits.

- **Learn how to cook** – I touched on this in the
intro, but trust me, you will eat cleaner for way
longer and be happier about it if you get creative
and explore ways to make the food you eat taste
delicious while still eating clean. There is this
defeatist mentality out there that all great-tasting
food is bad for you and 'clean' means 'tasteless'.
Not true! There are so many ways to cook the
usual suspects like chicken, fish and beef to keep
it interesting. There are so many types of cooking
oil now that are not only tasty but great sources
of essential fats and MCTs (medium-chain
triglycerides) like coconut oil, grapeseed oil,
virgin olive oil and many more. And it has never
been easier to find recipes. If you have a bunch
of ingredients in your fridge and you don't know
what to do, type them in on a search engine and
see if any recipes pop up, you'll be surprised
how often they do. I recommend stocking up
on herbs and spices and other seasoning, as
that can often be the difference maker. Plus,
many herbs and spices have health benefits; for
example, cayenne pepper is often associated
with fat loss which is why it is often an ingredient
in many fat loss supplements.

- **Limit your sodium** – While I'm all about adding a
little flavour with seasoning, and don't shy away
from salt and pepper, I do realise that you have

to be careful about your sodium (salt) intake, especially with the amount of food I eat in a day in comparison to a regular person.

For a long time, people have been just focused on sodium intake in the diet. This is because sodium is known to draw water from cells (this is why it is used as a preservative, as it dehydrates unwanted organisms on food) and the result is the body holds on to water. But actually, the more important factor is the sodium to potassium ratio. Basically, your cells act like a pump, and for every two potassium molecules that go in, three sodium molecules are pumped out. This affects fluid balance, which is our main focus here. Unfortunately, food companies are only required to print the sodium levels in their food, not potassium. Contrary to the belief of many who try to cut out salt completely, you actually need sodium to maintain a healthy water balance, but it's about moderation. Aim to eat sodium and potassium in equal amounts (the average American eats five parts sodium to one part potassium). Try not to add too much extra salt to your diet, try to consume potassium from quality fruit and vegetables, especially try to replenish potassium after a workout, and avoid big fluctuations in sodium intake and you should be just fine.

- **Eat natural: avoid processed** – Processed food may be the biggest double-edged sword in food history; the original motivation behind food processing was to preserve food and in fact dates back centuries. Very noble. Modern food processing techniques stem from the need to preserve food for soldiers at war, which is again very noble. Unfortunately, once the techniques became more and more refined, people realised that it could lead to huge profits (follow the money!), because by making food that lasts longer, you can make and sell more of it and offer the selling point of all selling points: convenience.

Let me clarify something before I continue; when I use the term 'processed food' I'm referring to food that has been *chemically processed*. Any food that has been prepared in some way or altered from its original form (for example ground meat) is technically 'processed'. What do I mean by chemically processed? Instead of real, whole food, food that has been made using a combination of refined food ingredients and artificial substances. Here's an example: People love to throw around the phrase 'whole grain' like it implies something healthy. But the reality is that most 'whole grain' products are those grains pulverised into flour then mixed with a bunch of chemicals. If I brought you a bowl of flour and a bowl of chemicals and asked you if it looked appetising, you'd probably look at me like I just asked you for your kidney. Getting a clearer picture now?

Here's a rundown of why to avoid processed foods:

— They're usually high in sugar and/or high in fructose corn syrup; if diabetes, heart disease and cancer don't concern you (!?!?) perhaps getting fat does.

– They're often full of refined carbohydrates; see above.

– They're a cocktail of chemicals; pick up a food item that you think might qualify as processed. Read the ingredients. If the ingredients list reads like a science exam, or if there are more ingredients that you don't recognise than ones you do, put it down. Ironically, 'diet' bars are often some of the worst offenders.

– They're low in nutrients; yes, sometimes companies will add synthetic vitamins and minerals to replace the ones that were lost during processing. If you think that's going to get you where you want to be I have a car with no wheels I want to sell you.

– They're often high in trans fats or processed vegetable oils; cheap fats from hydrogenated vegetable oils like seeds and soybean are just about the worst thing you can put into your body. Eat them if you want a significant increase in risk of heart disease, *the most common cause of death in Western countries today*. The excess of omega 6 acids also causes inflammation, the most underrated risk in health. Elevated inflammation is a risk factor for the most common disease of ageing. Worse than that, chronic, low-level inflammation is linked to diabetes, heart disease, cancer, depression and even Alzheimer's. If you want to learn more I recommend going to InflammationFactor.com.

— They require less energy to digest; because processed foods are a cocktail of blended food bits and chemicals, they don't require a lot of chewing or digestion, which means you eat more of them, and burn less energy digesting them. Next stop, Fat City. Population: you.

— They have less fibre — fibre basically keeps everything moving through your system. It also slows absorption of carbohydrates and feeds the good bacteria in the intestine. Think about it like this: If I left a turkey burger out all day, or even three days, then offered it to you, would you eat it? No? Well if you're not getting enough fibre that three-day-old burger is stuck to your insides somewhere.

— They're 'hyper-rewarding' and can be addictive. This is where it gets really evil. The human body is an amazing piece of technology; we're equipped with all kinds of awesome tools including taste buds, which help us navigate our natural food environment. We gravitate towards sweet, salty and fatty because we instinctively know these foods provide nutrients we need to survive. So food companies engineered food that is all three and therefore very desirable. When we eat them, our brains are so overwhelmed by the rewarding sensation of the food because we've never come across anything like this naturally. Our bodies have a mechanism from the brain that regulates energy balance, basically telling us when to eat and when to stop, and therefore keep us healthy. These foods bypass that mechanism because they're 'hyper-rewarding' and that leads to overconsumption. But that's not the worst of it...

The hyper-rewarding nature of this food can cause a dopamine release (dopamine is one of the most important neurotransmitters in the brain, associated with bodily functions and behaviour. If you want to know more please look it up) and essentially hijack your brain chemistry and make you 'addicted' to the feeling. There have been numerous studies that show that sugar and hyper-rewarding junk food activate the same areas of the brain as *cocaine*. Actual addiction of anything is often down to an individual's brain chemistry, but I bet if you think hard enough, you know at least one person who eats junk food regularly, almost systematically, without concern. I really believe that they have, in a unique way, become addicted to the hyper-rewarding nature of engineered processed food.

Master your Macros

In art and dream may you proceed with abandon. In Life may you proceed with balance and stealth – Patti Smith

The term 'Macros' has really come into fashion in the fitness realm in recent years, despite the fact that it has always been an established key to achieving your body goals. Macros is just an abbreviation of *Macronutrients*, referring to protein, carbohydrates and fat. Typically, when people are talking about their macros, they are referring to the ratio of protein to carbs to fats and the amounts of each they need based on their size and their current goals.

Here are the typical ratios. Keep in mind that these are not exact ratios that need to be followed religiously, as everybody is different and there are a number of other factors that affect your results. But in most cases, with good quality training, these are your typical ratios:

Mass Gain: Higher Carb – 40-60% carbohydrate, 25-35% protein and 15-25% fat.

Maintenance: Medium Carb – 30-50% carb, 25-35% protein and 25-35% fat.

Fat Loss: Lower Carb – 10-30% carb, 40-50% protein and 30-40% fat.

If you remember my point in the EAT Principles about understanding the relationship between carbohydrate and insulin, you'll see that the key factor that changes the most when it comes to diet is the number of carbs. If the thought of measuring everything is daunting, it shouldn't be, and I'll be the first to admit that I rarely measure exact amounts anymore, because I have developed a pretty good instinct of how much protein, carbs or fats something contains from just looking at it.

But in the beginning, the easiest way to develop this instinct is to remember the ideal principle of consuming at least one gram of protein per pound of bodyweight (a little more if you can) and then working out your other macro amounts as a ratio. For example, if you weigh 200lbs and you're in a mass gaining phase, if 200g of protein is 25% of your diet, 480g carbs would be 60% and 120g fat would be the remaining 15%.

Obviously, this ratio is a basic breakdown of what has proven to be effective for athletes over years of trial and error. But it's still a very simplified version of the right advice. This is under the assumption that you're going to divide those amounts of macros up over good quality sources. I mean, the 200lb athlete can't drink 200 grams of whey protein, eat 400 grams of sugar and 120 grams of butter and expect to add quality mass!

Protein

In the EAT Principles, we covered the essential information about why you need quality protein and the process it goes through in your body to serve its purpose as the building blocks of life.

Although there are differing schools of thought on the subject, a common consensus among the athletes and gym rats that I have encountered is that the best way to make use of the protein you consume is to take in somewhere around 30 to 40 grams at one time (based on an average sized male; I tend to aim for around 50g per meal). This is to allow the body to assimilate the protein effectively without too much being wasted. I should point out that there have been some very credible studies that suggest that the assimilation was not significantly affected by splitting it up over five or six meals or taking it all in one go. One such study is described in Tim Ferris' excellent book *The 4-Hour Body*. But from my experience and from the testimony of the superstar bodies that I know, 30-40 grams per sitting seems to work best (it also avoids overeating, which can cause the stomach to stretch and affects the shape of your waist.)

Here we will break down the most popular sources of protein from real food (protein supplements will be covered in the supplements section):

Eggs: Excellent source of protein; high biological value, low carb, good source of essential fats (whole eggs). Five large whole eggs will provide you with just over 30g protein on average. If you're trying to eat less fat and doing just egg whites, approximately eight egg whites will give you the same amount of protein. I always preferred whole eggs for the good fats and vitamins and minerals you get from the yolks. If I'm trying to lean up for a shoot or a special event I will switch to egg whites for a short time.

Chicken: Chicken has always been a popular choice in the physique realm and for good reason; 4 ounces of grilled, skinless chicken breast will provide your 30g protein, zero carbs and 5g fat. Eating roasted chicken, particularly with the skin on or the dark meat will provide higher fat content. Chicken is also a great source of potassium.

Tuna: A staple of my diet when I was a starving wrestler, tuna is good quality protein and very affordable. It has been one of the most popular choices among bodybuilders and physique fanatics for a long time. There are different types of tuna, but a 5-ounce serving of skipjack tuna (in water) will provide around 30g protein, zero carbs and almost no fat at all. My personal favourite is albacore (white) tuna, it has a slightly meatier texture and is not so harsh and fishy tasting. Tuna is also a good source of selenium, an antioxidant mineral that prevents cellular damage and is beneficial to your immune system.

Beef: There's nothing like a good hunk of red meat, and beef is the king of the reds. But there is a greater amount of discrepancy when it comes to eating beef as the nutritional content varies a lot depending on the cut. A lot of people tend to limit their red meat intake or avoid it altogether. That's their prerogative, more power to them. I personally eat quality red meat and always felt like I benefited from it. There are so many cuts to choose from when it comes to beef; my advice is to stick to leaner cuts but honestly, I'll chow down on a good rib eye quite frequently, I just make sure that if I'm eating a fattier cut, it's during a low-carb day. The saturated fat and cholesterol found in a good quality – preferably grass-fed – piece of beef is beneficial to hormone production, especially testosterone in men. Beef also provides a great amount of iron and is a real food source of creatine (approximately 4 to 5 grams per kg) which improves the work capacity and size of your muscles (covered in detail in *supplements*); a 4-ounce serving of lean ground beef (lean mince) will provide just over 30g protein and 8-10 g of fat.

Pork: The pigs seem to get left behind when it comes to the fitness world; pork is usually passed up for beef, chicken or fish. But occasionally pork can have its moments. There are lean cuts available like pork steaks. On average, a six-ounce serving of pork steak will provide your 30g protein and around 18g fat. Pork tenderloin can be very lean; in fact, ounce for ounce it contains less fat than chicken. Choose wisely and pork can be very beneficial in your quest for lean muscle. Oh and did I mention that pork is delicious? Obviously be careful with bacon and ham, as the sodium and nitrates are not on the healthy side. But in limited amounts they are fine, especially during low-carb periods.

Turkey: When it comes to low fat, turkey may be the undisputed champion of the lean meats. Obviously very similar to chicken, a 4-ounce serving of grilled skinless breast will give you your 30g protein and virtually no carbs or fats. If you insist on being calorie-conscious, this serving will give you just 120 calories.

Vegetarian Options: 6 ounces of Tempeh, a soy product, will give you around 30g protein, 20g fat and a good amount of magnesium, iron and vitamin B6. ¾ block of Extra Firm Tofu (also made from soybeans) will provide around the same protein and fat and is a complete protein (contains full range of essential amino acids). Peas provide about 8g protein per cup, making them a good accompaniment to a primary protein source. Quinoa provides about the same amount of protein as peas except it contains all nine essential amino acids. Nuts and nut butters are a good source of protein and good fats but go for natural options like natural peanut butter which gives you 8-10g protein per 2 tbsp serving. Beans are a great option; two cups of kidney beans will provide around 25g protein, and most beans (white, black, pinto etc) will do around the same. Chickpeas (used in hummus) have a high protein content (about 15g per cup) and again provide a good accompaniment.

The key to achieving a positive nitrogen balance on a vegetarian diet is to match up your proteins and consume them together so that you give yourself the best combination of amino acids so that the maximum amount of protein can be utilised by the body.

Controver-SOY: Tofu and other soy products have long been the go-to for vegetarians and have even been touted as a health food to carnivores. But the ugly truth about soy is that the majority of soy products consumed in the United States and Western Europe are not healthy; in fact they can be downright scary. In the US, 90 per cent of soybeans grown are genetically modified, which, in animal studies, showed an increase in allergies, sterility and birth defects. Most soybean crops are also covered in chemical herbicides. But that's not the worst of it.

First of all let me squash this myth; soy will not increase oestrogen in men. A few years ago, bodybuilding magazines (and I would bet manufacturers of whey protein) pushed the idea in fitness magazines that soy increased oestrogen so it was a bad idea for bodybuilders to use soy protein. This is not true; there is no evidence to my knowledge that suggests that male hormone levels are directly affected by soy consumption. However, soy has been known to affect hormone levels in women due to potent 'antinutrients' according to Dr Joseph Mercola who wrote for *Huffington Post*: "Just two glasses of soy milk daily provides enough of these compounds to alter a woman's menstrual cycle."

So what are antinutrients? Well, to be brief, they are a lot of hard-to-pronounce compounds like soyatoxins, phytoestrogens and saponins that wreak havoc on your body in a number of ways including reducing absorption of vital minerals, interfering with digestion, disrupting your endocrine system, blood clotting, toxicity, blocking of thyroid hormone synthesis and more which can lead to fun stuff like infertility, thyroid cancer, stunted growth in children, hormone imbalance and more. Sounds almost unbelievable, right? Something marketed as so healthy to be so damaging? The problem is that most of the soy products produced in the Western world are **unfermented** which leads to these problems, as the fermentation removes many of these harmful properties. **Fermented** soy from organic soybeans is not only a good protein source but has high levels of Vitamin K2. Tempeh, listed above, is an example of a fermented soy product, along with Miso and Natto. Tofu is NOT fermented, neither is soy milk or soy protein powder. In my opinion, it's not worth the risk.

Carbohydrates

I don't want you to think that just because I explained the importance of the relationship between carbohydrates and insulin, and what that means for your body, that I am anti-carbs. Nothing could be further from the truth, but I do feel that a lot of people approach carbs in the wrong way. For example, I don't believe in the traditional meal structuring of one protein, one carb and one veggie for every single meal. For one or maybe two meals that's acceptable, but most people don't need that many carbs throughout the course of a day and I believe that most people are just eating a few too many carbs overall.

For athletes and people looking for their superstar body, carbs are an important part of the diet; they are the body's preferred energy source and are going to help you perform at your highest level while you strive to gain lean mass, strength and shape.

We've already covered the amounts of macros, including carbohydrates, that generally tend to work for most. But I strongly reiterate that everybody is different, so play around with amounts and see what works for you. I never used to vary my amount of carbs that much, and when I finally did, I realised just how effective it can be, particularly for losing body fat. But simply thinking about the amount of carbs is not enough. You have to understand the difference between *simple carbohydrates* and *complex carbohydrates*, and when is a good time to consume each. You will also have a better handle on your diet and your body if you understand the basics of the *Glycemic Index*.

Simple Carbohydrates are carbs that are absorbed quickly and easily. Your body can use these almost immediately in many cases. Simple carbs spike blood sugar quickly, which means the energy from them is not sustainable and whatever doesn't get used is stored as fat. To conclude, the optimum time to consume simple carbs is either a small amount during your workout or immediately following your workout.

Complex Carbohydrates take longer to digest and don't spike blood sugar as drastically, so can often provide a better form of sustained energy. In many cases, complex carbs also contain a higher amount of fibre than simple carbs, which is important for maintaining digestion, nutrient absorption and fat loss.

But in recent years, we have also developed an understanding of a characteristic of carbs that goes beyond the notion of just simple and complex. This is known as the *Glycemic Index*, or GI. The GI has helped determine the rates at which carbs are released into the bloodstream. When this system was introduced it showed that certain carbs which were thought to be complex actually absorbed more quickly than some that were considered simple.

Rather than deciphering carbs which are simple, complex, low GI or high GI, I've combined the information and tried to simplify it and given you a list of *slow carbs* and a list of *fast carbs*:

Slow carbs: Oats, sweet potato, nuts, legumes, brown rice, quinoa, pasta, dairy products, nuts, fructose from apples, pears, plums, peaches, grapes, oranges and grapefruit, vegetables (except root veggies).

Fast carbs: Sugars, honey, potatoes, bread (especially white), white rice, flaked or puffed cereals, instant oatmeal or grits, carrots, corn, peas.

To summarise: adjust your amount of total carbs based on your macro needs determined by your goals, then aim to consume mostly slow carbs, saving your fast carbs for after your workout to replace glycogen quickly, aid transport of amino acids and nutrients to your muscles and aid recovery (and growth). If you stick to this general principle and adjust as you go forward, you will be in control of your energy levels, muscle growth and body fat levels.

Fats

In *The EAT Principles* I explained why good fat is so valuable and so misunderstood. Essential Fatty Acids (EFAs) are so important for healthy heart function, vitamin and mineral absorption requires fats and so does your cellular energy. However, because when it comes to nutrition labelling we are still fairly basic and simply state the amount of 'fat' in a food, the bad fats have besmirched the good name of the heroic fats out there.

When I professed the evil of processed food one of the things I touched on was the presence of hydrogenated vegetable oil, easily one of the worst things you can eat on a regular basis. This is an example of a *trans fat*.

Trans fats have two types: *Naturally occurring trans fats* that are produced by some animals, and subsequently are found in small amounts in some animal products like meat and dairy. The real villains are the *artificial trans fats,* created in an industrial process that adds hydrogen to vegetable oils hence the term 'hydrogenated'. The main source of trans fats in processed food is 'partially hydrogenated oils'. To give you an idea of how much you should be avoiding these, the US Food and Drug Administration (FDA) made a preliminary determination in November 2013 that these fats are no longer *Generally Recognised as Safe (GRAS).* Trans fats are used because they're cheap, and the companies that use them don't care about you or your body. Trans fats raise your bad (LDL) cholesterol and lower your good (HDL) cholesterol, increase your risk of heart disease and stroke and, oh yeah, they make you look and feel like crap. Check labels, particularly on packaged food products, for hydrogenated oils as they can be lurking in foods marketed as healthy. Generally, trans fats are most prevalent in the following foods:

- Processed foods
- Fast food
- Deep fried food in commercial locations, as the oil used can be used over and over again...nice.
- Cookies, crackers, cakes etc.
- Margarine and other non-butter spreads.

Saturated fats in moderate amounts can be beneficial to your physique goals and to your health. Contrary to popular belief from decades of misinformation, saturated fats are not the enemy. Dr Jospeh Mercola, *New York Times* bestselling author, wrote:

> *"A misguided fallacy that persists to this day is the belief that saturated fat will increase your risk of heart disease and heart attacks. This is simply another myth that has been harming your health for the last 30 or 40 years.*
>
> *The truth is, saturated fats from animal and vegetable sources provide a concentrated source of energy in your diet, and they provide the building blocks for cell membranes and a variety of hormones and hormone-like substances."* – Taken from *7 Reasons to Eat More Saturated Fat* on www.Mercola.com

A healthy dose of saturated fat will keep your brain functioning correctly, as well as your lungs and liver. The important factors when it comes to using saturated fats to building your superstar body are improved nerve signalling; where saturated fats essentially act as messengers for your metabolism and aid insulin response, and hormone production, particularly in men. Testosterone is the be-all-end-all when it comes to giving you what you need to have a great body as a man: more muscle, less fat, more strength, more energy and more sex. Sound good? Well, you need cholesterol to produce testosterone and you get that from saturated fat. The best examples of good saturated fats are:

- Organic grass-fed beef and dairy products (full-fat) from grass-fed cows

- Coconut oil, MCT oil, palm kernel oil (all examples of medium-chain triglycerides*)
- Brazil nuts

Medium-chain triglycerides (MCTs) have been shown to help excess calorie burning, are the most readily available fat for energy and promote fat oxidation. When consumed in place of carbohydrates, they can be especially effective in improving your body composition.

Unsaturated fats are generally considered the healthiest fats to consume. The two types are monounsaturated and polyunsaturated. Both kinds have been shown to improve blood cholesterol levels. Look for unsaturated fats rich in Essential Fatty Acids, particularly Omega-3. While you can get EFAs from plant sources, the body most easily converts the EFAs found in fish.

- Fish sources: salmon, trout, herring, tuna, mackerel, sardines
- Plant sources: avocado, flaxseed, olive oil, nuts.

The Good, the Bad and the Great – I've devised this system when it comes to fats because, let's face it, not all of you have the time or the patience to be researching which foods are good sources of saturated, unsaturated, monounsaturated, polyunsaturated and essential fats. So instead I've broken it down into three groups:

Bad. *Avoid as much as possible*: vegetable oil, fast food, hydrogenated oils, processed food, deep-fried food.

Good. Eat in moderation: grass-fed beef, butter and dairy from grass-fed cows, organic ghee, natural nut butters.

Great. Eat frequently, particularly during low-carb periods: coconut oil, cacao butter, avocado, salmon and other fatty fish, extra virgin olive oil, flaxseed, chia seeds, almonds.

Eating Habits

By now, you've probably realised that I strongly believe in figuring out what works best for you and you alone, so these are by no means rules to follow. But when it comes to your diet, eating habits can play an important role as well as what you're actually eating. I'll cover some of the more frequently discussed diet techniques in this section.

How many meals? – The amount of macros you consume will be determined by your goals, size, body type and physical demands. But how you break up your total macros over a day can often be debated. I can tell you from my own experience, I've always trusted my instincts, eaten when I'm hungry or when I feel like I need to and usually that results in eating about five times per day which seems to be the case for most of the superstar bodies I know. I sometimes just eat four meals, and I know some people who break up their protein, carbs and fats over six, seven or even eight meals. It depends on how big your appetite is, your lifestyle and how you train. My best advice is to have a good idea in your mind at the beginning of the day and eat accordingly.

If you know you're going to be busy, maybe you eat bigger and less frequently. If your appetite isn't as strong as usual, eat small and graze through the day. The most important thing is to hit your macros number, especially protein.

Breakfast – Most people are getting breakfast all wrong. They eat a load of carbs either in the form of processed high GI cereal, toast or they eat slow carbs under the impression that it will give them sustained energy throughout the day. This is a fundamentally incorrect approach and I'll explain why.

For a long time breakfast has held the title of 'The Most Important Meal of the Day' and there is a lot of validity to that argument. When you think about it, it's really just common sense; you haven't eaten anything while you've been asleep, so depending on when you last ate the night before, you are probably in the range of eight to ten hours without food by the time you wake up. Not surprisingly, your body is at its least anabolic (muscle-building) and at its most catabolic (muscle-wasting) after sleep. So the most important thing is to consume some quality protein ASAP. Eggs are the obvious choice, but if you don't have a big appetite in the morning, a whey protein shake is fine too. But that's only one part of the breakfast equation...

As I said, the majority of people chow down on a load of carbohydrate because they've been told for years that you need it for energy, especially those angelic 'whole grains' that are supposed to give you long-lasting energy. Have you seen the commercial with the girl who works at the coffee shop and after eating her frosted mini-wheats she's remembering all her orders and firing on all cylinders? Yeah, that might be the case at 10am, but by 11 that wheat and sugar is sending her into a crash; primarily because they're simple carbs, but also because after you've gone hours without eating, you have in many ways 'reset' your body, which can often be a good thing if you eat the right stuff after fasting. Like I mentioned before, your body is the most advanced piece of equipment you own, continuously evolving and adapting to input and environment. When you eat breakfast, you are essentially 'programming' your metabolism for the rest of the day, telling it what to rely on for energy. If you start with fast carbs or even slow ones, you are programming your body to rely on carbs for energy. So if your goal is lean, full muscle and low body fat, you are better off programming your metabolism to use fat for energy and preserve muscle with quality protein and good fats.

A small amount of low-GI carbs is OK too, but my personal technique is to wait until later in the day to consume some low-GI carbs and I feel less bloated and more energised by doing high protein and high fat in the morning. I also understand that some people are busy, especially in the morning, so it might be a good idea to get some low-GI carbs. I also usually train in the afternoon, so if you are a morning trainer, some carbs might be a good idea.

My typical morning is a small whey protein shake (I use Bulletproof Upgraded Whey from grass-fed cows with added MCT powder) followed by four whole eggs, lean bacon or turkey bacon and half an avocado. I drink a cup of Bulletproof Coffee with Grass-fed Butter and Cacao Butter.

What to eat Pre- and Post-Workout – This is a subject that has really evolved over the years since the 'golden age' of bodybuilding in the 1970s. In that era, many of the best bodies in the world including Arnold and Frank Zane (my two all-time favourites) believed that food should not be consumed either too close to a workout or too soon afterwards, based on the idea that the body needs blood to be pumped to the muscles and eating will cause blood to go to the stomach and intestines for digestion instead. Remember that back in those days, a lot of focus was on maintaining a slim waist and not stretching the stomach, and let's face it, if you look at pictures of Arnold and Frank in their primes, they knew exactly what they were doing. I always say that you can't argue with results, so I take heed of this advice. Nowadays, a lot more emphasis has been placed on the importance of your post-workout nutrition; some fast-absorbing carbs and all-important protein to replace glycogen stores, prevent muscle breakdown and start the rebuilding ASAP. From research and years of my own experience and that of many top athletes and superstar bodies, I've concluded that the popular amount of post-workout carbs seems to be around one-third of a gram per pound of bodyweight.

In other words, divide your weight by three and that's the amount of carbs you should aim for post-workout. So in my case, at around 250lbs, I aim for about 80g carbs after an intense workout. Protein-wise, about half the amount of carbs seems to be best, so in my case, around 40g. There is a lot of evidence to suggest that there is a 15- to 20-minute window of time to consume some nutrition before muscle breakdown occurs. So combining the advice of the classic era and of the modern era, I tend to drink a post-workout shake containing quality protein (whey) and fast carbs (dextrose, maltodextrin) about 15 minutes after my workout, to allow the blood flow to return to normal a little bit, but avoid muscle breakdown. I don't follow this religiously, however, as there are times when I'm carb cycling and keep carbs as low as possible. On those days, I'll make sure that the small number of carbs I do eat are post-workout, but I increase my protein. Once again, experiment and see what works best for you.

Pre-workout is another key area. I personally have always felt better if I have some kind of food in me before I train. It should be adequately digested if you eat at least an hour before training. I tend to go for protein, good clean fats for sustained energy and strength plus, depending on what I'm doing in my training session that day, maybe some slow carbs. A good example would be a turkey sandwich on whole wheat or rye bread, with avocado and spinach.

NEVER train on an empty stomach, not even cardio in the morning, which is a popular but short-sighted approach. Many people have often done empty stomach cardio under the impression that the body will burn fat for energy as there is nothing else to use. In fact, muscle glycogen is more readily available than fat, so you will likely lose muscle first before fat. If you're a fat-loss fanatic, you should at the very least consume some protein before your early cardio. But in credible studies, it has been shown that people who consumed a small amount of carbs oxidised just as much fat as those who did not when performing low-intensity cardio.

Carb Cycling – I mentioned before that carb cycling is my weapon of choice when it comes to reducing body fat. I am what is known as a 'hard gainer', someone who struggled mostly with adding quality mass but found it relatively easy to stay lean due to being primarily an ectomorph. When I was first starting out, I needed a huge amount of calories and protein to add bulk to my slight frame. Even in my first few years in wrestling, I was wrestling so often that I had to eat so much just to keep my size. As a result, carb-consciousness was never something I really needed to think about. I would hear people talk about low carbs and I would see guys on the road with me ordering no carbs and I would think, "I'm glad that's not me." I would attempt low carb diets if I was attempting to get lean for a photo shoot or something like that, but would always be frustrated at how I lacked fullness in my muscles and started to look 'flat'. Then I learned about carb cycling.

The premise of carb cycling is to gradually empty your body of carbs over a short period, to encourage the body to oxidise fat for energy during exercise and to maintain a good level of insulin sensitivity. This is then followed by a short period of higher carb intake, to replenish glycogen and glucose, avoid muscle breakdown and maintain good energy levels. Like I said, I have found this to be the happy medium between limiting carbs to be lean and cut but not lose muscle size and fullness.

A typical carb cycle looks something like this: three days of low carbs, decreasing daily e.g. Day 1: 100 grams, Day 2: 75 grams and Day 3: 50 grams or less followed by two days of higher carbs e.g. Day 4: 100 grams and Day 5: 200 grams.

My personal carb cycle is shorter. I employ two days of low carbs followed by one day of moderate to high carbs.

The key to getting carb cycling right is to eat clean, quality carbs: not sugars (except post-workout and fructose from real fruit) and not processed carbs. I also don't count fibrous veggies in my carb count, as the fibre is more important for digestion and fat loss, and their effect on insulin is minimal. Experiment with your individual carb cycle and see what works for you; the best way to do this is to keep track of it with a nutrition diary.

Controlled Fasting aka Intermittent Fasting – This eating technique focuses on going for a prolonged period without eating (or eating a very small amount of protein or raw vegetables) and then returning to a 'feeding' period for a shorter period of time. It follows the same kind of principle as carb cycling, but focuses on entire calorie intake rather than just carbs. The idea is that fasting allows your cells to empty and refresh, making you more receptive. The fasting period is also supposed to maximise the Sympathetic Nervous System's "fight or flight" response and promote alertness, energy and fat burning. Conversely, the short feeding window which usually involved eating a lot in a short period at night, is supposed to engage the Parasympathetic Nervous System's ability to promote calm, relaxation and digestion through deep sleep, which also promotes better growth and repair. There are different methods including the popular *Warrior Diet*, *LeanGains* and *UpDayDownDay* among others.

I wouldn't recommend fasting for everyone, but if you have a particularly hectic lifestyle and can be prepared with good quality nutrition for the feeding periods, then you may benefit from the technique. I have also heard several accounts of men experiencing greater benefits from controlled fasting as they get into their late 30s and 40s and their metabolism slows down and appetite decreases. Try it and see how your body responds.

Carb Back-Loading – *Carb Back-Loading* follows along the same lines of principle as Carb Cycling but over a shorter period of time and with a more drastic carbohydrate binge. To start, go about five days of little to no carbs, 30 grams or less daily. After that, eat little to no carbs during the day until around 5pm then after your workout, go crazy; eat any and all carbs, particularly high GI carbs to replenish glycogen and use insulin to your advantage, as insulin will store carbs in your muscle cells while leaving fat alone if these carbs are consumed immediately after resistance training. The key to making carb back-loading work is to train hard in the mid to late afternoon. If you train in the morning, this protocol probably isn't for you. I enjoy using this technique during a mass gain phase, where I'm trying to gain quality mass and my appetite is high, especially in the colder months. It also gives you a little more freedom with your diet, enjoying starchy carbs like potatoes, breads, even pizza etc if you really hit the gym hard.

There is another version of the same protocol known as *Carb Nite* (both carb back-loading and carb nite have been covered and pioneered by John Kiefer. Visit www.carbbackloading.com or www.carbonite.com for more information and to buy the books).

Carb Nite is a longer version of back-loading. In a nutshell, you go about ten days on little to no carbs; again try to aim for 30g or less. This essentially recalibrates your system to use fat for energy. Keep starches to a minimum. After ten days, Have a 'Carb Nite'; from about 5pm you can throw caution to the wind and eat all the carbs you like, fast or slow. The ten days recalibrating changes enzyme production and makes it highly unlikely for you to gain fat from one night of craziness. After that you repeat this technique but with a shortening time frame; enjoying one carb night per week and eventually if your body allows, even one every three to four days.

Supplements

Superstar Spotlight: Rob Terry

Nutritional supplements are essential: to be used in the right places within a diet to maximise the body's needs for nutrition under great physical demands such as intense training.

Timing is everything and makes all the difference between a supplement plan that works and one that doesn't.

My choice of supplements are:

• A fast-acting whey isolate protein for after training and occasionally after breakfast.

• Amino acids while I am training and small amounts throughout the day to help keep the body from breaking down muscle tissue.

• Carbohydrate and creatine supplement for after training.

• Taking a good brand of multivitamin complex is important along with cod liver oils and joint support supplements.

These are the supplements that have been a staple in my diet.

Even though supplements are important to a diet, they are a **supplement** to a diet. There is no replacement to eating quality foods loaded with nutrients. To me eating solid food makes the difference between my body looking good or looking great!

Rob Terry is a fitness model, bodybuilder and pro wrestler. He has in my opinion one of the most incredible drug-free bodies in the world. He looks like a Clydesdale horse! For the six years I've known him, he has always been shredded and loaded with dense, full muscle. He has devoted his life to the pursuit and science of bodybuilding and developing a great physique.

There is no doubt that diet and training go hand-in-hand to create a superstar body. And an effective diet should also be enhanced by the enormous range of nutritional supplements that are available today. But I must emphasise the point made by Rob in the above passage: never lose sight of the meaning of the word supplement. They are an enhancement to a good diet, not a safety net for a bad one. There are a plethora of products out there that promise the earth, but usually just cost it. I'm going to attempt to give you a good idea of what to look for.

Protein Supplements

Whey Protein – The king of all nutritional supplements, whey protein should already be a part of your daily intake. Whey is the watery portion of milk that separates from curds when making cheese. It is then converted into a powder form. This technically makes it a milk protein, although the separation removes the lactose, which makes it a popular replacement for milk for people who are lactose intolerant. However, the reason it has become a staple of athletic diets is the high Branched-Chain Amino Acid (BCAA) profile and the extremely high Biological Value (BV). BV refers to the value that measures how well the body absorbs and utilises the protein, converting it into nitrogen which the body can retain and use for lean muscle growth. Whey protein's BV is 104, followed by egg protein at 100. Whey protein is also absorbed extremely quickly, which makes it ideal to consume immediately after a workout, when you need to restore the nitrogen balance and supply amino acids to the muscle fibres that were just torn and need to be rebuilt. I always consume whey protein after a workout with some kind of fast-absorbing carbohydrate like a sports drink, vitargo or fruit, so the aminos can be transported and glycogen can be restored.

Key points: High Amino Acid profile and Biological Value (BV). Fast absorption which makes it ideal for post-workout.

What to look for: Whey from grass-fed cows. Whey concentrate or isolate. Added colostrum for growth and immune system boost. Filtered using proprietary filtration and drying (many proteins are dried at high

temperatures which destroys the components).
What to avoid: Proteins with fillers that cut costs for
the manufacturers: hydrolyzed, ion exchanged, micro or
cross-flow filtered. These processes denature the original
proteins.

Casein Protein – Often an overlooked protein, casein is another milk protein that I recommend that you introduce to your diet. While the BV is lower than whey (77) the key benefit to casein is that it has a deliberately slow absorption rate, providing a steady supply of amino acids. This makes it particularly useful before bed, when you go without muscle fuel for hours. The first protein I ever bought was a box of cheap calcium caseinate when I was 12 years old; I had no idea at the time what I was doing, but looking back it probably helped as my metabolism was so high at the time that the steady stream of aminos helped me build lean muscle quickly. Studies have also shown that casein consumption elevates metabolic rate through the night, aiding fat loss. It also increases satiety, making you less prone to cravings.

Key Points: Longer lasting absorption. Increased metabolic rate overnight. Increased satiety.

What to look for: Micellar Casein rather than Calcium Caseinate. Micellar is the truer form or slow-digesting casein, although Calcium Caseinate is much more affordable and still effective.

What to avoid: Fillers and unnecessary carbs, especially if you plan to consume before bed.

Collagen Protein – A relatively new breakthrough in the market, but something I use regularly, collagen is great for healthy soft tissue repair. It provides particular proteins that promote cohesion, elasticity and regeneration of skin, cartilage and bone (you have probably seen collagen advertised in skincare products for anti-aging). Collagen facilitates the synthesis of creatine, great for muscle-building. It also makes the building blocks of connective tissue more bioavailable, enhancing flexibility and strength. I use a flavourless collagen and add it to my whey protein after a workout. It also provides proline (great for cartilage) and glycine, which aids neurotransmission (yes, your brain needs protein), motor sensory pathways and ATP synthesis.

Key Points: Regenerates skin, joints and bone. Aids creatine synthesis. Supports brain function.

What to look for: Easy-mixing, genuine collagen.

What to avoid: Formulas that only contain a small amount of collagen.

Soy Protein – The long-term health risks of *unfermented soy* have already been covered, so it should come as no surprise that soy protein supplements remain a constant source of debate in the health and fitness world. Soy protein has become the go-to protein source for vegetarians, vegans and the lactose intolerant, especially those who wish to improve their physiques. However, there has been a lot of controversy as to the alleged health benefits of soy, which seem far-fetched at best. In retaliation, many health publications have published reports about the negative property of soy protein consumption. Looking at soy protein (in particular, concentrate and isolate) from a purely physique-benefitting perspective, I tend to think that soy is ineffective for the price. It has a low BV (74) despite the fact that it technically provides all essential amino acids, making it a complete protein. In my experience, it has also been hard to mix and has a mealy, chalky taste and texture. That's not something I want to put myself through. If you are vegetarian or vegan and want to keep soy in your life, I suggest you use soy sparingly and in addition with other protein sources. Take the time to do some real, impartial research, as vegetarians need to work hard to get the full spectrum of nutrition for building their bodies. You're going to want a good blender too. If you're lactose intolerant, use egg protein, and almond or cashew milk are alternatives that in my opinion taste better.

Key Points: Suitable, cheap alternative to animal protein for vegetarians, vegans and lactose intolerant.

What to look for: Fermented soy protein. Well-rated soy protein isolate and concentrate for taste.

What to avoid: Cheap soy products, they most likely contain glyphosate, chemically engineered to withstand heavy doses of herbicides.

Egg Protein – A somewhat overlooked contender in the protein division, egg protein is another good choice for your everyday protein supplement. As we already discussed, egg has a very high BV and contains all eight essential amino acids. It's a very good choice for people who don't respond well to whey and contains no lactose. The major issue I've encountered with egg protein among peers and through my own use is that the mixability isn't great and the taste is also below the standard of most whey products.

Key Points: High BV, lactose-free alternative to whey protein.

What to look for: Easy-mixing, well rated in taste tests.

What to avoid: Low-rated formulas, formulas with fillers and high amounts of sugars.

Beef Protein: A relatively new arrival on the protein market, beef protein isolate is being offered by a couple of brands, marketing it as a supplement with all the benefits of lean beef (high protein, creatine, BCAAs, zinc) in a convenient powdered form. After conducting some further research, it appears that the product consists mainly of gelatin. In other words, all the pieces of the cow that get thrown away after the butcher is finished like joints, hoofs, ears etc. This ground-up surprise then gets fortified with BCAAs and creatine and they have a powder that they can legally market as beef protein. Suddenly not as empowering as the vision of downing a sirloin steak in two gulps. The jury is still out, but for the money, I'd stick to whey.

Creatine

Many in the fitness world and bodybuilding community consider creatine the most important supplement perfected and manufactured with the exception of whey protein.

In a nutshell, creatine is a nitrogenous acid that supplies energy to all cells in the body, particularly muscle cells. Creatine encourages water to be held in muscle cells which allows them to perform for longer, which is why it was popularised by both endurance athletes and bodybuilders when it first made an impact on the scene in the 1990s. The first high-profile athletes to be named as users of creatine supplements were British athletics stars Linford Christie, Colin Jackson and Sally Gunnell (God Save the Queen!).

The implications on muscle endurance have diminished over the years due to several studies that show creatine to have a significant effect on high-intensity short-term muscle power, but not a significant effect on intra-exercise synthesis of creatine phosphate in the body. So in other words, it will aid your strength and power, not your endurance. So if you intend to train hard and leave it all in the gym, then creatine is definitely going to help you. More good news for guys; studies on athletes including rugby players and college football players have shown that testosterone and Insulin-like Growth Factor-1 (IGF-1) levels increased significantly with the combination of creatine consumption and resistance training.

Creatine also improves cognitive function and memory, so if the idea of bigger and stronger muscles doesn't convince you to regularly take creatine, maybe better brain power will.

There are a number of different types of creatine but the most common are creatine monohydrate and creatine ethyl ester (CEE). Monohydrate is the long-established form of creatine supplement, and is basically creatine complexed with a water molecule, usually in a powder form. CEE has been touted to have better absorption than monohydrate, but no peer-reviewed studies conclusively prove this claim. So it seems that supplement companies perpetuated this idea to charge a higher price for CEE. Stick with creatine monohydrate. Combining creatine with fast carbs will increase creatine muscle stores, which is why there are a lot of products on the market that are a ready-mixed combination of creatine and fast carbs. Consuming creatine and carbs post-workout is a great idea. But on a daily basis, I'd recommend taking 3-5g of pure creatine with water.

BCAAs

Branched-Chain Amino Acids, usually referred to as BCAAs, are a supplemental form of the amino acids that are most important for muscle repair and maintenance. Once a highly touted product, BCAAs became less fashionable as products like pre-workout formulas, fat loss formulas and test boosters started to steal their limelight. This was bad news for BCAAs but worse news for you, the aspiring superstar body. Why? Because BCAAs have a ton of benefits and frankly, should be high on your priority list when it comes to supplements.

If you don't know by now, amino acids are essentially the building blocks of muscle construction. They have long been known for their ability to aid an athlete with a high protein diet increase their muscle mass. What many people don't think of however, is how important BCAAs are for people who are trying to shed body fat. Have you ever attempted to lean up for the summer by dieting, then become frustrated by looking flat and soft? Chances are your diet made you catabolic – your body broke down muscle for energy and on top of that, your reduced energy intake will also slow protein synthesis. In other words, you lost muscle and your body can't rebuild it. This is where you really need BCAAs; they increase protein synthesis and even improve the cellular activity that carries out protein synthesis. They also reduce protein and muscle breakdown.

Many top authorities on the subject including Charles Glass, legendary trainer of top athletes and IFBB pro bodybuilders, are proponents of consuming BCAAs during training (intra-workout) because they believe that strongly in the importance of preventing muscle breakdown. I personally keep a tub of BCAAs in my car at all times so that I can take some just before I walk into the gym and as soon as I come out.

My conclusion: BCAAs are not that expensive, and if you intend to train hard and want a hard, full body, then they should be on your shopping list. Look for a BCAA product with a high amount of *Lutein*. Always aim to get the full spectrum of aminos from food and whey protein, but BCAAs make sure that hard work doesn't go to waste. Before, during and after training are all good times to take BCAAs as well as upon waking and before bed. When you're on a low-carb diet or reduced calories, increase your BCAA intake to avoid losing your hard-earned lean mass.

Fat Loss Supplements

The market is flooded with diet pills and fat loss formulas that all promise to torch your body fat in as little as one month, despite not including any instructions on how to eat and train and instead implying that simply taking these pills will do the job. If you believe that, I feel sorry for you.

The majority of fat loss formulas contain the following key ingredients: *Caffeine, Green Tea, Cayenne Pepper* and *L-Carnitine*. The rest is made up of 'proprietary blends'; in other words, 'a bunch of stuff we don't have to be specific about'. Do you want to regularly ingest pills that contain a mystery mix of God-knows-what? Didn't think so. My advice: save your money, don't buy the over-priced fat loss products. Instead, if fat loss is your primary objective, buy the key ingredients individually, they will last longer and give you more fat loss bang for your buck.

Caffeine: Caffeine has long been established as an aid to fat loss. It kick-starts the process of lipolysis, which is the body releasing fatty acids into the bloodstream (in other words, using fat for energy). Caffeine as we all know is also a stimulant, which improves mental and physical performance, which means you have a better chance of maximising your minutes in the gym. Pure caffeine pills are very affordable too, and easily available (when I was in the UK I preferred *Caffeine Pro* from MyProtein.com and here in the States I use *Smart Caffeine* by *Natural Stacks*.) 200mg seems to be the effective dose of pure caffeine, but if you're sensitive, start with 100mg. Pure is much different than caffeine as part of an energy drink. Also please be aware that caffeine is a stimulant and do not use it if you are under the age of 18, pregnant or suffer from heart conditions or other conditions that make you high risk. Consult a doctor before starting if you are unsure.

Green Tea: Green tea has been used for centuries in Asia as a digestive, and has become popular in Western culture with good reason; it's packed full of beneficial compounds such as tannins (astringents; they shrink tissues and contract structural proteins), catechins (antioxidants that provide more antioxidant power in one cup than a serving of broccoli, preventing free radical damage after workouts), flavonoids (protection against infection) and theanine (an amino acid that acts as a natural tranquiliser).

Green tea is a popular fat loss agent as it raises resting metabolic rate without any of the negative aspects of stimulants (jitters, decreased appetite, irritability). Theanine is also calming mentally but doesn't impair you physically, which can actually aid performance and focus in my experience. The important thing to remember is to buy good quality whole-leaf green tea and invest in a steeper or infuser (I use a single serve infuser ball, it's so easy and cheap.) The stuff in bags is not nearly as effective or pure.

Cayenne Pepper (Capsicum): Cayenne is another health ingredient with a long history. It has reportedly been used as an herbal supplement since the 17th century. The key component of cayenne is also the reason for its heat, capsaicin. Capsaicin may help the immune system, improve circulation but more importantly for this discussion, increases body heat and metabolism. The most effective way to supplement it is either in powder form (with water and lemon juice) or capsules. There are very dedicated sources for information for all the other reported health benefits of cayenne, the most comprehensive of which is www.cayennepepper.info.

L-Carnitine: Acetyl L-Carnitine (sometimes referred to as ALCAR) is the popular supplement form of

L-carnitine, often categorised as an amino acid but actually a cross between a vitamin and amino acid formed in the liver and kidneys but stored elsewhere, mostly in muscle. In real food, its best source is red meat, but can also be found in avocado. L-carnitine helps you transport fat into cells to be oxidised (used as fuel) especially during intense exercise. Without enough L-carnitine, dietary fats can't be used as fuel, so it is important you get an adequate supply and the easiest way to ensure that is by supplementing it. There has also been a lot of research to suggest it can enhance insulin's actions on muscle cells, so it is advisable to take with your post-workout meal too, in order to aid recovery. Don't go overboard; high doses have resulted in rare cases of nausea, cramps and diarrhoea. If you have a sensitive stomach, tread carefully.

Good news for guys, some studies have even suggested that L-carnitine can aid erectile dysfunction, probably because it boosts blood flow. I recommend taking it in a pure powder form with some high-GI carbs either during or after your workout.

Stick with these key compounds and your fat loss and performance will get a boost plus your wallet will be grateful; for the price of one month's supply of some of the leading fat loss supplements out there, you could buy each of these individually in much greater amounts.

Pre-Workout Formulas

One product line that has really made a big impression on the scene in the last ten years is the pre-workout. If you have ever shopped online or walked into a sports nutrition store, or even most pharmacies and supermarkets these days, you have likely seen products promising "Huge Pumps" or "Max No2" and so on. Within my generation, I've seen pre-workouts evolve from a fairly specialised product to something that many guys now consider an essential. Vanity is a powerful thing; I've been on the road with guys who have asked me, "Bro, do you have a scoop of pre-workout I can borrow? I hate training without pre-workout."

I should point out that for the most part, pre-workouts actually do exactly what they say they're going to do, which is probably why they're so popular. They will increase your 'pump' (when blood is forced into the muscle and gives a full, tight look and feel) and they will increase your energy with stimulants. But just like fat-loss cousins, they can be over-priced for what you get, and they all contain the key ingredients which, if you buy separately, will give you what you need and save you ingesting fillers or mystery 'proprietary blends'. It will also save you money.

Arginine: The most important component of a pre-workout is the amino acid arginine. It converts in your body to nitric oxide (NO) which allows your blood vessels to expand so more blood can reach your muscles. This is for 'show' and for 'go'; increased blood also means increased oxygen and nutrients to your working muscles. There are different types of arginine, the most common being *L-Arginine* and *Arginine Alpha-Ketoglutarate or AAKG* (try saying that one fast). They have slightly differing profiles but as long as you're getting these two you are on the right track.

Citrulline: Citrulline converts to arginine when ingested. And the general consensus from research and trial-and-error is that a combination of citrulline and arginine is more effective than either individually.

Caffeine: We've already covered the benefits of caffeine in the fat-loss portion, but pre-workout products tend to feature caffeine anhydrous, which is a drier form of caffeine and is considered best for increased energy and strength. It should also be noted that caffeine can help reduce 'the burn' – the perceived pain of resistance training.

BCAAs: I've already sung the praises of BCAAs but pre-workout, the important ones are *Leucine, Valine and Isoleucine.*

Taking a combination of these supplements about twenty minutes before a workout will give you all the pump, focus and protein synthesis you need, without the jitters of caffeine mixed with sugar and the hot flush of Niacin, commonly featured in the pre-workout formulas. Much like my advice for fat-loss supplements, this route will also save you a lot of money in the long run.

Vitamins

Hulk Hogan encouraged kids to say their prayers and eat their vitamins, and while I'm going to leave the subject of religion well alone, I will say the Hulkster was dead right about the vitamins.

Vitamins are one of the longest-reigning supplement champions, but are not without debate; you may recall a certain sensational story that received a lot of traction in mainstream media in 2013 claiming that vitamins are a waste of money! The reason this story got so much traction is because it was written by an editorial panel of doctors. Everybody should trust doctors, right? Well...

Doctors actually receive little to no class work on nutrition or dietary supplements, so anything they know about the subject is based on what they've learned on their own, not at medical school. But that's not all; this article ("Enough Is Enough: Stop Wasting Money on Vitamin and Mineral Supplements" *Annals of Internal Medicine*) was based on just three studies, which were very cherry-picked (selected based on having the right evidence to support their claims) while there are multiple studies conducted over multiple years that demonstrate many benefits to vitamin and mineral supplements.

So why would these doctors go out of their way to besmirch vitamin and mineral supplements? Call me a cynic, but I'm going to use my favourite motto when trying to find the truth: *follow the money*. This study, despite being slanted science at best, was covered in a lot of mainstream media. Mainstream media often has close associations with political parties, political parties rely on big financial donors including pharmaceutical companies (Barack Obama and Hillary Clinton are the top recipients of donations from the pharmaceutical industry, and in 2004 the Bush campaign received over half a million dollars from drugmakers, according to *The Center for Responsive Politics*). For pharmaceutical companies to make money, people need to be sick. Could it be that increased vitamin and mineral consumption was causing too many people to be healthy and eating into the pharmaceutical industry profits? I'll let you make up your own mind.

We've focused a lot on minding your macronutrients, so it's time to look more closely at *micronutrients*. Making sure you get a good dose of these daily will facilitate proper body functioning, which will allow the processes you are encouraging your body to perform to keep running smoothly. Think of it like this; if your macros are the gasoline, the micronutrients are the oil.

Let's start with the basics; take a high quality multivitamin supplement every day. There are some that are geared more towards men or women. This is fine if you want to take one of those, I just try and make sure that the multivitamin I take is 'food rich', preservative- and gluten-free. This is a helpful tip; many supermarkets now have a 'whole food' or 'natural food' section. I tend to get my vitamins from this section as they are usually organic and contain fewer fillers.

A good multivitamin will cover all your bases, but here are a few vitamins and minerals that have some extra benefits and may be advisable to take individually if you want a superstar body:

- Vitamin A (aka retinol): Healthy vision, immune system improvement from mucous membrane development, bone growth.
- B Vitamins: Specific B vitamins serve different purposes but all pertain to breaking down and using food to its full potential. Get a good B vitamin complex containing B1 (Thiamine) B2 (Riboflavin) B3 (Niacin) and B12 if possible.
- Vitamin C: Antioxidants protect from free radicals and benefit immune system function. Maintains connective tissue in cartilage and tendons.

- Vitamin D: Absorption of calcium and phosphorous, ensuring bone health. Aids increase in testosterone for men (Vitamin D3)
- Zinc: Immune system, increased ability to fight infection, improved protein synthesis, bone health, increased testosterone in men.
- Magnesium: Improved IGF-1 production, allows melatonin and serotonin production for better sleep and relaxation, cleanses bowels of toxins, improved enzyme function.
- Potassium: Muscular strength, improved blood pressure, metabolism, water balance.

Nootropics

Sometimes referred to as smart drugs or neuro enhancers, nootropics are a group of drugs, nutraceuticals, supplements and food sources that improve one or more aspects of mental function like attention, memory, focus or motivation. For the purpose of this book I'm focusing on the supplements and nutraceuticals (if you're wondering what nutraceutical means, it basically means the same as supplement, but rather obviously is a combination of the words 'nutrition' and 'pharmaceutical'). Nootropics are still a relatively new market in various stages of research and development but are nonetheless making a big impact. Some common nootropics include *Ginseng, Ginkgo Biloba, Isoflavones, Choline* and *Bacopa Monnieri*.

Superstar Spotlight: Ben Hebert

Two deep breaths.

I glance up at the clock.

Two minutes left.

I'm down by seven points. The wrestler facing me down across the mat brought a strong game plan today, and hasn't missed a beat. He's taken me down again and again. My stomach lurches. I think about how I should have spent more time working on my sprawl. He hits another double leg and slams me down to the centre of the mat. Somehow he lands in my full guard. He could just ride this out and stall for the win, so I loosen my legs, hoping he'll pass.

In an overconfident moment, he grounds one of his arms on the mat. I latch on as fast as I can and throw up a sloppy Hail Mary of a triangle. Before he can posture up, I clamp down and begin to squeeze. I need to cut off his oxygen and force him to tap out. My coaches start yelling, "Grab the leg! He's trying to pass!" He's going for a basic escape, something I've countered a hundred times before. But not this time. I don't move with him. I don't flow. My mind and body are working against each other.

He escapes the submission.

Moments later the ref is holding his arm up, and he's walking away with the medal I came here for.

That fight was a defining experience for me.
I was devastated. In the following days, I thought about everything but how I lost. I just couldn't face it. After putting off going to training again for weeks, I realised I had to get it together. For me to get better, and win the next bout I entered, I needed to work through that failure and learn the lessons it held for me. I'd spent thousands of hours on the mat. I'd won plenty of bouts before. I knew that on skills, I was more than capable of beating that guy.

It was my mind that came up short that day. I didn't have the confidence, focus or motivation to get the job done.

To get better in my pursuits I knew that I needed to work on my mental performance. When that clicked, I immediately shifted my focus. I wanted to develop a routine that would make me unbreakable.

THE UNFAIR ADVANTAGE
Supplementation is not a cure-all. It's not a magic solution that makes you better than everyone else. But a good supplementation routine can give you an edge. It can definitely bring your natural strengths to the fore, and can absolutely enhance your ability to perform.

In my quest to improve my mental capacity, I found that there was a whole community of people dedicated to optimising their mental performance. They had experimented extensively with nootropics, and had made some impressive discoveries.

Nootropics – also referred to as cognitive enhancers or smart drugs – have been used for millennia. Just about every ancient culture references nootropics in one form or another. They're safe, proven and effective. **They were the edge I was looking for.**

Soon I was talking to Abelard Lindsay, a living legend in the nootropics community. He shared with me a stack he'd called CILTEP, an all-natural combination of artichoke extract, forskolin and Vitamin B6.

CILTEP was a game-changer.

It increased my ability to focus on the task at hand. It made me motivated and able to deflect distractions more effectively. My mind was sharper, and my thoughts came more quickly and fully formed.

When I was training, my mind and body got in sync. I was acting as soon as the thought entered my head. I was able to think a couple of moves ahead, and didn't get thrown off my game as easily if something unexpected happened.

The changes I experienced with CILTEP led me to start Natural Stacks.

Being able to pinpoint exactly which compounds were working for me was remarkable – I was able to experiment with various combinations until my performance was at an all-time high. You see, most supplement companies are very protective of their ingredients and formulas. While they might give you *an increase in performance, you don't know what the active ingredient is that's making all the difference.*

This is problematic for two reasons. Firstly, it removes your autonomy in the situation and ties you to that company. Secondly, and even more importantly, everyone's brain chemistry is a little different.

While most people see similar results from most stacks (combinations of nootropics), you need to be able to experiment with different ingredients at different concentrations in order to work out what is most effective for you.

That's why Natural Stacks is an open source company. We want to enable you to make the right choices for your body and brain, rather than acting like everyone is exactly the same.

When you're researching and experimenting with supplements – whether nootropics, protein powders and BCAAs, creatine or vitamins or minerals – keep in mind that your body is unique. Each supplement has a unique purpose and will yield a unique result. What works for your friend or favourite celebrity trainer may be just as effective for you, but don't be surprised if it's not.

The key to optimising your mental performance – to truly sharpen your mind into that of a champion – is to always be seeking. Ask lots of questions. Delve into what makes you uncomfortable. Do the hard work and find what truly works for you, what drives you, what gives you the edge that puts you ahead.

Ben Hebert is an entrepreneur, startup specialist, international speaker and co-founder of Natural Stacks (www.naturalstacks.com) as well as a Brazilian jiu-jitsu enthusiast and self-confessed foodie. I thought I was fairly accomplished for my age until I met Ben, who makes me feel lazy. He is one of the smartest people I know and has a refreshing ethical approach to supplements: tell the people exactly what they are taking. This is why I was so eager and proud to become associated with both Ben and Natural Stacks.

My Typical Meal and Supplement Day

I'm currently holding at around 250lbs and my abs are visible. I'm pretty happy with this composition. Obviously I'm always striving to improve; adding mass to certain areas, improving definition in others, but for the most part, I'm in a maintenance phase. So my focus is split between quality muscle maintenance, fat oxidation, mental clarity and healthy testosterone levels. Keep in mind that my preferred method of carb control is carb cycling, so on days 1 and 2 (lower carbs) my carbs may consist of only post-workout carbs, or slow carbs before and fast carbs after my workout, then on day 3, I would enjoy some starch with my evening meal like potatoes. With that in mind, a typical day for me looks something like this:

Upon Waking: 2 large scoops whey protein w/ water. Bulletproof coffee w/2 tbsp grass-fed butter, 1tbsp cacao butter, 1tbsp collagen protein, cinnamon, half cup of almond or cashew butter.

Supplements: Vitamin D3, Krill Oil, CILTEP. 20-30ml Apple Cider Vinegar w/ water*

Mid-Morning: 5 whole eggs, 5 rashers turkey bacon, half an avocado

Supplements: Multivitamin, Niacin (non-flush kind) BCAAs

Midday: 6 oz chicken breast OR steak, 3 large celery sticks, 3 tbsp natural peanut butter

Afternoon: (approx. 1 hour before workout): 2 cups cooked oats w/ milk and cinnamon.

Pre-Workout: BioCreatine™ (Creatine w/Himalayan salt), 200mg caffeine, B Vitamin complex, BCAAs, arginine.

Post-Workout: 50g whey protein, 50-60g fast carbs e.g. dextrose or similar. 3-5g creatine

Evening: 8 oz chicken/steak/salmon/pork, portabella mushrooms, baked potato, fibrous veggies e.g. broccoli, spinach, asparagus or similar.

Night: 2 scoops whey protein w/ 2% milk, 1tbsp natural peanut butter, chia seeds, flax seeds, MCT oil and mixed berries (strawberries, blueberries and raspberries)

Supplements: Vitamin D3, Magtech ™ Magnesium, Potassium, Zinc

Apple Cider Vinegar is a natural cleanser that has been used for centuries. It kills bad bacteria but most importantly, it reduces blood sugar levels by improving insulin sensitivity. This helps prevent unwanted fat gain from elevated insulin levels.

Obviously I rarely eat the exact same thing every day but when I am at home (not on the road wrestling) this would be a very typical day. It gives me around 300g quality protein, tons of good fats and limited carbs but all at good times depending on whether they are fast or slow. I split my supplements up through the day to allow maximum use and digestion, and I find I'm more defined when taking a potassium supplement at night to counteract any sodium I've consumed throughout the course of the day and prevent water retention. The D3 in the morning and at night, combined with a good supply of healthy fats and arginine, plus zinc and magnesium at night, helps my testosterone production.

This is a way to show you how I implement my own advice. Tweak it to suit your own needs and your size, body type and goals.

Part 3

LIVE

I am not a product of my circumstances. I am a product of my decisions – Stephen Covey

The mantra of this book is the mantra I try to live by every day: Train. Eat. Live. After fifteen years of trial-and-error, reading, discussing and experiencing ways to make my body better, I realised that the main reason I would hit obstacles and plateaus along the way was that I was only focusing on the first two. Today, with a career in a cutthroat industry, bills to pay, physical and emotional demands of my profession and son to provide for, I have a much healthier balance that I believe has me geared towards greater success and happiness in whatever I choose to do.

Although this section will be much smaller than the previous two, I don't want you to take it for granted; the amount of words should not imply their importance. I just wanted to share with you some of the things I feel are important outside of training and diet that help you achieve the superstar body you desire, whatever that body is.

Recovery Techniques

You need to recover after you exercise. You know that already, but you're not really interested. 'Recovery' is one of those words that people throw around that is safe and sensible, but it's not exciting. It's like 'insurance'. You know you need it, but you hate buying it, hate dealing with it and couldn't be less excited if you tried. Recovery techniques don't provide you immediate satisfaction; you can't feel it working like you can when you have a pump after lifting weights, or the satiety after eating something when you're hungry.

I want to stress to you the value of expedited recovery: not the *importance* of it, but the *value* of it. If I tell you it's important, you'll accept it but it won't change the way you look at it. Hopefully if I stress the value of it you might change the way you look at it. Think of your recovery techniques as earning interest on an investment: Your training and diet are your investments, and your gains are the interest you earn on them. But that interest is earned over time; by improving your recovery, you're placing a condition on your investments that reduces the time it takes to earn some interest and ultimately, see a return on your investment.

Stretching

Superstar Spotlight – Kurt Angle

Many people, including Nick, have asked me what it is that keeps driving me to bust out another workout, to push myself again and again after everything I've done in my career. I think that the biggest thing I've learned throughout my career is "If you don't use it, you lose it." So if I don't train as hard as I can today, I can't do the things I love to do.

I've had many injuries that are well documented, some of them so severe that for all intents and purposes I shouldn't have come back from them, but I did. So when I did, I always made myself train as hard as I did before the injury, so I could still be the best I can be. Today, I'm 46 but some days I feel like I'm 100! Other days I feel like I'm in my twenties, but regardless of how I feel, I push myself to train as intensely as I can. And I hope that people can take heed of this advice: whether you're an athlete or simply someone trying to stay in shape: the harder you push yourself, the younger you keep yourself.

One of the things I see is people who say they used to exercise and now live a sedentary lifestyle and they say they can't get back into it. They can, but many won't because the motivation has taken a huge hit. Because after you've quit exercise, you're most likely going to be able to do less than you did before, so stay active, always.

I'll be honest, the numbers I hit in the gym today are nowhere near the numbers I used to hit, but it doesn't matter, because I'm going the hardest I can go, and it's getting me where I need to be. I'm happy and grateful to be able to do that.

The biggest thing I've learned later in my life is the importance of flexibility; I'll admit that I never really focused on it during my amateur career or even prior to the Olympics, but I can't believe how much career longevity I've gotten out of doing more stretching. It's been able to not only prevent further injuries but help my existing ailments heal and improve. It's another way I've been able to keep myself at the top level, keeping up with all these guys in their prime.

Live Long to Live Long: I was in Dallas, Texas at the College Park Arena for a pay-per-view event and after my match with Jeff Hardy, I had a session with Dr Tim Adair who we all refer to as "Dr Tim", who was our resident chiropractor. I kept suffering from a nagging pain at the bottom of my neck and it turned out to be a muscle restriction. After adjusting me, Tim said, "Man, your traps have grown since I last saw you, hope you're stretching them properly." I said, "How do I stretch them 'properly'?" Tim went on to explain how people who lift weights frequently develop all this tension in their traps which is restricting nerves from receiving messages freely. He also told me all kinds of anatomical stuff about how important it is to stretch for a variety of reasons. In a nutshell, there are all kinds of important things in that cervical area of the spine that I'm not qualified to talk about, but Tim advised me to hold a dumbbell of decent size (I use 75lbs) by my side and stretch the opposing trapezius muscle by leaning my head to the side opposite the side holding the weight. It really stretches the traps and the feeling is awesome. I started following his advice and within two weeks I had gained another half inch on my traps from nothing but stretching! Needless to say I have continued with his practices and am now working on applying the same quality stretching to all my muscle groups. Tim reinforced my understanding of how much longevity you will gain from stretching, and his mantra that I remember every time I perform that trapezius stretch is "Live Long to *Live Long.*"

Stretching has evolved a great deal, especially in the last decade. For a long time, *static stretching* (holding stretches for a sustained period, usually between 10 and 30 seconds) was the go-to 'warm-up' technique. I remember every football practice would involve stretching before we got started. Luckily today we have realised that static stretching as a warm-up activity is fundamentally wrong, as the muscles need to actually **be warm before they are stretched**. Stretching muscles that are not yet warm and without the pliability required can actually be highly detrimental and stretch the connective tissues, weakening them when they need to be at their strongest. But there is no denying that stretching allows a feeling of greater mobility and range of motion, so what's the answer? Enter *dynamic stretching*; warm-up exercises that involve movement with fast bursts of a stretch on the muscles, generating heat, encouraging blood flow and allowing a more limber feeling. Better still, dynamic stretching ahead of your workout or practice challenges your balance, coordination and body awareness, activating your mind and body to perform optimally. Popular dynamic stretches include high kicks, arm swings, twisting lunges, high knees, trunk twists and chest expansions.

The beauty of dynamic stretching is you can take almost any conventional stretch and create your own sped-up version to make it a dynamic stretch. I personally rely heavily on dynamic stretching before I train legs or any power training, and especially before I wrestle, doing a lot of leg swings and high kicks to warm up my hip flexors, lower back and hamstrings so that my mobility is there in the ring, especially given the fact that with boots, knee braces and knee pads, some of that mobility can be limited. A great website for dynamic stretches is www.brianmac.co.uk/dynamic.htm

Static stretching is something that needs to take place *after* you train, or just at home in your free time, but make sure you generate some heat first. Your muscles are warm, pliable and your circulation is high. Static stretching will condition your connective tissues, making sure they keep up with your muscles as they strengthen and place a higher demand on those connective tissues. What if your primary concern is just looking good? You don't have to worry about stretching, right? Wrong. Stretching improves the way your muscles look.

Muscle has what's called a fascia (*myofascia*), which is basically a skin around the muscle itself, which is very strong and is designed to limit how much a muscle belly can grow so it retains its shape and structure. That sounds bad, and to a lot of size-obsessed guys it is, but the fascia is important, because to achieve a great-looking body, you want to obviously increase the size of the muscle belly, but you also want to retain the shape, so the objective is to gain the maximum size without losing shape and therefore aesthetic quality. Stretching allows you to retain the shape, resulting in clean sweeping lines of separation and allowing your muscles to flow into one another, giving that all-important chiselled look. If you don't stretch, enjoy that blocky 'carrying pillows under both arms' look that nobody likes whatsoever. We've all seen 'that guy'. Don't be that guy.

Yoga or Pilates are both excellent ways to maintain flexibility and improve the look and condition of your hard-earned muscle. It challenges you to put your muscles to the test, resulting in further cuts, separation and density. Yoga and Pilates both focus on balance. Balance = Symmetry. Symmetry = Attractive body.

Hot/Cold Therapy aka Contrast Therapy

A few years ago I read an article about Russian athletes and their coaches, and how back in the 1960s especially, their training techniques and innovations absolutely smoked the rest of the world. So did their knowledge and understanding of anabolic steroids, by the way, but that's another story. In actual fact, their pioneering of anabolics is in many ways what led their coaches and physicians to explore and perfect many of the advanced recovery methods used today. Anabolics increase strength, muscle size and aid muscle recovery and hypertrophy (the increase in size volume of muscle fibres due to enlargement of cells) but it happens so quickly compared to a drug-free environment that risk of injury increases. This is why those coaches were focused more heavily on recovery techniques. After reading the article I became much more interested in researching and experimenting with proven recovery methods and without question one of my favourites is contrast therapy, also known as hot/cold treatment.

You may be familiar with hot/cold treatments if you have suffered any minor injuries of muscles or joints like a sprain or strain. In recent years, contrast therapy has become the popular effective method recommended by doctors and physical therapists due to its ability to relieve pain and inflammation. Research, trial and error from trainers and strength coaches over the years has also concluded that heat causes a mild sympathetic stimulus that basically fires up your body's *adaptive mechanism* without the need for physical stress on the body. In other words, exposure to heat kick-starts the recovery process and tells the body "start rebuilding now". Heat also opens up blood vessels, allowing blood flow and a supply of nutrients and oxygen to the target area. Conversely, cold exposure slows down blood flow to the area, reducing pain and inflammation. This is why with hot/cold treatments you should always **start with heat and end with cold**. The only exception might be if you're trying to sleep immediately afterwards, in which case slowly build back up to moderate warmth.

The easiest method to apply this technique is in the shower. I recommend doing this at least once a week, save it for after a particularly intense resistance day. The key to getting the most out of this method is to make the contrast as high as possible; as hot as you can bear it followed by as cold as you can bear it. Try to make each period of exposure between 1 and 5 minutes but remember, your body adapts to stimulus, so just like with exercise and diet, keep it varied each time so your body doesn't get used to it. If you train at a gym or health club that has a sauna, steam room or hot tub, these are all great methods to utilise too; apply the same principle, transitioning between the heat and a cold shower. Hot tubs or Jacuzzis are more effective for the lower body as the shower heat is difficult to apply to the lower body. Repeat the process three or four times to get maximum benefit. You'll find that you will sleep really well after one of these sessions too.

Massage and Soft Tissue Treatments

Step into the 21st century with me and understand that massages aren't just for couples on vacation or girls on a spa day. Massage and soft tissue treatments significantly improve your recovery and the quality of your musculature. Just like stretching, massage, particularly deep tissue, causes myofascial release, expanding and loosening the muscle fascia allowing for greater growth and increased strength. Massage treatments also improve circulation which I believe plays a big part in longevity, especially for people who lift weights. Tissue work releases toxins that build up in some areas, so make sure you drink plenty of water after soft tissue treatments of any kind (you will need to pee a lot).

I'm not an expert in this area, but I know a thing or two about improving your body, and part of that is trusting other experts when the time is right. Fortunately for you, there are tons of qualified expert massage therapists in the world, and if you're proactive and communicate with them, they will recommend all kinds of effective treatments that suit your individual characteristics and needs. These treatments include *Active Release Technique* (ART), *Myofascial Release*, *Muscle Activation Technique* (MAT) and *Active-Isolated Stretching* (AIS) to name a few. Finding a good therapist and undergoing some of these treatments whenever you can afford to (I usually do twice per month) will help you recover, prevent injuries, and make significant gains in a shorter period of time.

Low-Intensity Cardio

This is going to sound self-contradicting, as earlier I discussed the drawbacks with steady-state cardio. I stand by my words as they pertain to low-intensity cardio for a fitness tool. However, as a recovery tool, **occasional** low-intensity aerobic activity can be beneficial to regenerate cells, improve circulation and increase oxygen and nutrient delivery to your muscles. If my legs are sore after leg day (they always are) the following day I will often do some low-intensity recumbent bike, stair master or incline treadmill to get some blood pumping and I feel it helps. If you suffer an injury, aerobic work can speed up the healing process. Remember, blood flow = healing.

Salt Baths

Once again, it's time to check your stereotypes at the door because taking a long soak with certain bath salts can be an effective tool in speeding the recovery process, allowing you to get back to work in the gym sooner and make gains faster.

Epsom Salts, otherwise known as magnesium sulphate USP, draws toxins from the body when absorbed through the skin. When you exercise, you release more toxins into your system which need to be eradicated to allow maximum regeneration. Epsom Salts also reduce swelling and sedates the nervous system, which aids deep sleep, especially when combined with the cooling period after a hot bath. Add around 500 grams (two cups) or more if you can to a hot bath. You can also use Celtic or Tropical Sea Salts, which also help draw impurities from the skin as well as relieve aches and swelling because of the high magnesium content.

Electronic Muscle Stimulation (EMS)

If you want to really push the boat out and are willing to spend the money, then investing in an EMS machine may be something to consider. EMS machines provide differing levels of pulsating movements to muscles in a localised way and provide the same benefits as massage; increasing blood flow and therefore oxygen and nutrients to muscles, and facilitating removal of waste products and toxins allowing maximum regeneration. They can be useful for people with busy or sedentary lifestyles outside the gym, for example if you have to be at a desk a lot.

The Sense and Science of Sleep

Sleep is the golden chain that ties health and our bodies together – Thomas Dekker

There is so much more to sleep than most people realise. Our health, our minds, our ability, our productivity and therefore our success, relationships and happiness all rely on a steady supply of ZZZs. Unfortunately, many of us still have a profound lack of understanding when it comes to what the difference between good quality and bad quality sleep is, and the implications of sleep when it comes to our lives, especially if one of your goals in life is to have a superstar body. Let me point this out right off the bat: Muscle growth and fat loss both depend on sleep. If you're under the impression that less sleep means losing weight, you're right, but it's muscle you're losing, not fat.

As a pro wrestler, I have had to deal with an almost crippling lack of sleep at times, which is one of the reasons I developed such a keen interest in sleep science; I started researching how to make the most of the limited sleep time I get on the road sometimes. Here's one of the roughest examples: After flying from the East coast of the US and landing in Dublin, dealing with the five-hour time change, wrestling that night, getting back to the hotel at 1am physically exhausted but riding high on adrenalin from the show, waiting for room service, trying to get to sleep at 2am knowing that the bus leaves for the airport at 6am sharp, and... I can't sleep. That sucks.

First things first, let's address snoring; if you snore every night it may be harmless but it may be a symptom of sleep apnoea. If you find that you get plenty of sleep but still find yourself feeling tired or drowsy during the day and you're a snorer, it may be worth seeing a physician because sleep apnoea is no joke. The pauses in breathing prevent air from flowing, depriving your blood of oxygen and therefore your heart, organs and brain. It can be treated easily and may save your life in the long run. Don't take regular snoring lightly. For more information and insight on all things sleep, visit www.sleepfoundation.org

I'm going to give you a few sleep terms and their definitions:

- REM – REM stands for *Rapid Eye Movement*. REM sleep is a stage of sleep when you do most of your active dreaming. It's called REM because it's characterised by fast back-and-forth movement of the eyes.

- NREM – No prizes for guessing that NREM stands for *Non-Rapid Eye Movement* sleep. Your body cycles between NREM and REM sleep. During NREM is when your heart rate drops and your body temperature decreases, preparing you for deep sleep, which is when the body repairs and regrows tissues, and bones, muscle and immune system are strengthened. Contrary to popular belief, 'deep' sleep is actually a period of NREM, not REM sleep. REM sleep is when your brain is more active, hence the dreams and eye movement.

- Sleep Homeostat – This is a [homeostatic] mechanism that regulates sleep intensity. It reacts to amount of activity and amount of sleep. In other words, how tired you are. The sleep homeostat enables organisms to compensate for loss of sleep.

- Circadian Rhythm – The circadian rhythm, sometimes referred to as *the circadian clock*, refers to the cycles of light and dark and the way your body reacts to it. The key component of this is when darkness causes the pineal gland in the brain to release *melatonin*, the body's sleep-inducing hormone.

I cannot stress enough the need for good quality sleep. Not just 'enough' sleep, enough quality sleep. If you're an average 21st century person, you're already messing with your circadian rhythm significantly every day with all the glare from TV screens, phones, tablets and computer screens emitting an unwanted 'blue light' that reduces the intensity of melatonin release in the brain or shuts it off altogether. If you're one of these people that 'needs the TV on to help them get to sleep', I'm afraid you're not providing your body with a lot of recovery during your sleep, and could be slowing your results down significantly, not to mention wearing down your immune system and decreasing your brain power. Attempt to limit your screen time at least two hours before you intend to go to sleep: not before you go to bed, before you intend to be asleep. Once you start to feel the difference, you will be encouraged to cut out time in front of a screen at all unless it's totally necessary.

You may notice in the previous paragraph that I referred to the time that you intend to go to sleep. If your response to that was "I don't have a time that I plan to go to sleep" then maybe you should consider it; research and case studies have shown that circadian rhythm benefits from definitive, regular times of waking and going to sleep. Sometimes, I will have a show within driving distance and jump at the chance to get home and sleep in my own bed (my king sized Tempur-Pedic is one of the best investments I ever made, even if it did cost more than my first two cars combined). After finally getting to bed at 2am or even later, I will look forward to sleeping as long as I want the next day, only to find that I will still wake up at 8am even without an alarm. This used to drive me crazy until I learned that this is in fact a sign of a healthy circadian rhythm and in some ways and indicator of a good sleep homeostat too. Start thinking about having a definitive time that you go to bed and wake up. However, it still doesn't change the fact that I didn't get enough quality sleep, so what's the answer? Naps.

I love naps. As of this writing, my son is seven months old and he still likes napping although he's already showing signs of discontent for the encouraged day siesta. I wish small children could understand just how much they will one day wish they could nap during the day when they are vehemently resisting. While kids may respond to a nap suggestion with a tantrum, I will gladly steal a short nap whenever I feel like I need it. I read about the Japanese approach to what we now refer to as 'power naps' and how many companies in Japan allow 15-minute nap breaks and have shown increased productivity as a result. I have been taking 15-minute power naps my entire adult life. I simply set a 15-minute timer on my phone (the phone screen is then shut off and I enable airplane mode) and I lay down, close my eyes and focus on allowing all my muscles and joints to relax. Sometimes I feel like I'm sleeping, sometimes I'm completely awake but whatever the case, when the time is up I simply get up and carry on. On rare occasions (like if I'm very sleep deprived) I may extend my nap in 15-minute increments, but never nap for more than one hour, as that is when you start to enter REM sleep which will affect your sleep that night and start a bad cycle.

Be like Ozzy: No, don't bite the head off a bat (or a dove) but be the prince of **darkness**. It's vitally important to sleep in as much total pitch-black darkness as you can. Get blackout curtains, block as many sources of light as you can, if you have to have your phone on, put it face down and away from your eye line. Cover or obstruct LEDs. All this will aid your circadian rhythm and improve the quality of the sleep you get. Remember, your muscle growth and fat loss both depend on sleep.

You need energy to sleep, not stimulants. This may sound obvious, but caffeine too late in the day will screw up your chances of good quality sleep. For most people, a 2 or 3pm cut-off is advisable at the latest. But food energy is required for good quality sleep. What you eat has a profound effect on how you sleep. Most notably, the presence of good fats, in particular omega-3s. The brain needs EFAs to function properly because the brain never sleeps, but it does call the shots. Make sure you consume some good fats close to bedtime. The brain also needs glycogen to function while you sleep, so depending on your physique and carb needs at the time, some clean natural sugars like raw honey or a small amount of fructose may be beneficial. You may recall in the Supplements section of EAT that some supplements I recommended improve sleep, the most notable being magnesium (I use Magtech™ by Natural Stacks as it contains different kinds of magnesium for full effect. I occasionally use GABA, a powerful relaxation agent. I wouldn't recommend it every night but maybe once or twice a week. Biohacking guru and big influence on yours truly Dave Asprey has written extensive advice on other ways to hack your sleep including some of these principles and many more in great detail. Visit www.bulletproofexec.com to learn more.

So to summarise:

- Little to no screen exposure (TV, computer, phone etc) two hours before bed until sleep.

- Try to develop a sleep and wake-up time routine

- Take naps to improve mood and productivity (never more than one hour)

- Be the prince of total darkness, no light = better sleep

- Supply your brain with the nutrition it needs to help you shut down: good fats, a little sugar and magnesium.

Goodnight.

Thank you for reading this book. It means a lot to me that even one single person would ask my advice, as I'm just as much a student of this game as any one of you reading this. A huge thanks to all the special men and women who contributed their superstar body philosophies and approaches for me to share with all of you.

We're all on a never-ending journey of self-improvement; there is no perfect body, no perfect state of health or performance. Yet millions of us all over the world love the thrill of the chase. But if I can impart one final piece of advice it would be this; don't sacrifice your enjoyment of life for a good body. Your superstar body is just the packaging of the entire product you are offering the world. Live a long, healthy, happy and accomplished life and let your superstar body be a part of it.

So the next time you see yourself and you realise you are now the person you admire, don't ask yourself "How do you train?" "How do you eat?"

Ask yourself,

"How do you LIVE?"

Glossary

Abduction – Movement of a limb away from the middle of the body.

Abs – Abbreviation for the abdominal muscles (Rectus Abdominus, Transverse Abdominus).

Accommodating Resistance – Increasing resistance as the lifter's force increases through range of motion. Nautilus machines are known for providing accommodating resistance.

Adduction – Movement of a limb toward the middle of the body, e.g. flyes for chest.

Aerobic Exercise – Prolonged, moderate-intensity exercise that uses oxygen at or below the level at which your cardiorespiratory (heart-lung) system can replenish oxygen in the muscles. Aerobic literally means 'with oxygen'. Common aerobic activities include running, cycling, swimming, dancing, and walking.

Agonist – Muscle directly engaged in contraction, which is primarily responsible for movement of a body part.

Amino acids – A group of compounds that serve as the building blocks from which protein and muscle are made.

Anaerobic Exercise – Exercise of much higher intensity than aerobic work, which uses up oxygen more quickly than the body can replenish it in the working muscles. Anaerobic exercise eventually builds up a significant oxygen debt that forces an individual to end the exercise session quickly. Anaerobic exercise (the kind of exercise to which bodybuilding training belongs) burns up glycogen (muscle sugar) to supply its energy needs. Fast sprinting and weightlifting are typical forms of anaerobic exercise.

Antagonist – Muscle that counteracts the agonist, lengthening when agonist muscle contracts.

Antioxidant – Small compounds that minimise tissue oxidation and help control free radicals and their subsequent negative effects.

Atrophy – The decrease in size and functional ability of tissue or organs.

Bar – The steel shaft that forms the basic part of a barbell or dumbbell. These bars are normally about one inch thick, and they are often encased in a revolving metal sleeve.

Barbell – Weight used for exercise, consisting of a rigid handle 5-7 feet long, with detachable weight discs at each end.

Balance – A term referring to an even relationship of body proportions in a man's physique. Perfectly balanced physical proportions are a much-sought-after trait among competitive bodybuilders.

Basic Exercise – A bodybuilding exercise which stresses the largest muscle groups of your body (e.g., the thighs, back, and/or chest). Typical basic movements include squats, bench presses, and deadlifts.

Benches – A bench is the long piece of seating equipment typically used for most exercises that are not performed standing. Most benches can be adjusted to be flat, inclined or declined.

Biomechanics – Science concerned with the internal and external forces acting on a human body and the effects produced by these forces.

Body composition – The percentage of your body weight composed of fat compared to fat-free mass.

Bodybuilding – A type of weight training applied in conjunction with sound nutritional practices to alter the shape or form of the human body. Also the name of a competitive sport where athletes are judged on the size and shape of their physique.

Buffed – As in a "finely buffed finish" – good muscle size and definition.

Bulking Up – Gaining body weight by adding mass in the form of muscle, body fat or both.

Burn – A beneficial burning sensation in a muscle that you are training. This burn is caused by a rapid build-up of fatigue toxins in the muscle and is a good indication that you are optimally working a muscle group.

Calories – The unit for measuring the energy value of foods.

Carbohydrates – Organic compounds containing carbon, hydrogen, and oxygen. They're a very effective fuel source for the body. The different types of carbohydrates include starches, sugars, and fibres. (Carbohydrates contain four calories per gram. Glucose blood sugar is a carbohydrate used by every cell in the body as fuel.)

Cardiorespiratory Fitness – Physical fitness of the heart, circulatory system and lungs that is indicative of good aerobic fitness.

Cardiovascular Training – Physical conditioning that strengthens heart and blood vessels.

Chalk Powder – Used on hands for secure grip.

Cholesterol – A type of fat that, although most widely known as a "bad fat" implicated in promoting heart disease and stroke, is a vital component in the production of many hormones in the body. There are different types of cholesterol: namely, MDL and LDL (MDL being the "good" form and LDL being the bad form).

Circuit Training – Going quickly from one exercise apparatus to another and doing a prescribed number of exercises on each apparatus, to keep pulse rate high and promote overall fitness.

Clean – The movement of raising a barbell or two dumbbells from the floor to your shoulders in one smooth motion to prepare for an overhead lift. To properly execute a clean movement, you must use the coordinated strength of your legs, back, shoulders, and arms.

Clean diet – This refers to eating nutrient-rich, low-fat meals.

Concentric – The lifting phase of an exercise, when the muscle shortens or contracts. For example, when you lift the weight in a bench press, pressing it from your chest to the lock-out position, that's the concentric, or "positive," phase of the exercise.

Crunches – Abdominal exercises – sit-ups done lying on floor with legs on bench, hands behind neck.

Curl-Bar – Cambered bar designed for more comfortable grip and less forearm strain.

Cut Up (or Cut) – A term used to denote a bodybuilder who has an extremely high degree of muscular definition due to a low degree of body fat.

Dead Lift – One of three powerlifting moves (other two are squat and bench press). Weight is lifted off floor to approximately waist height. Lifter must stand erect, shoulders back.

Deficiency – A sub optimal level of one or more nutrients that are essential for good health, most often seen with vitamins. A deficiency can be caused by poor nutrition, increased bodily demands (especially from intense training), or both.

Definition – The absence of fat over clearly delineated muscular movement. Definition is often referred to as "muscularity", and a highly defined bodybuilder has so little body fat that very fine grooves of muscularity called "striations" will be clearly visible over each major muscle group.

Delts – Abbreviation for deltoids, the large triangular muscles of the shoulder.

Density – Muscle hardness, which is also related to muscular definition. A combination of muscle mass and muscle density is highly prized among all competitive bodybuilders.

Diet – Food and drink regularly consumed by a person, often according to specific guidelines to improve physical condition.

Diuretics – Sometimes called "water pills," these are drugs and herbal preparations that remove excess water from a bodybuilder's system just prior to a show, thereby revealing greater muscular detail.
    Harsh chemical diuretics can be quite harmful to your health, particularly if they are used on a chronic basis. Two of the side effects of excessive chemical diuretic use are muscle cramps and heart ar-rhythmias (irregular heart beats).

Double (Split Training) Routine – Working out twice a day to allow for shorter, more intense workouts. Usually performed by advanced bodybuilders preparing for contests.

Drying Out – Encouraging loss of body fluids by limiting liquid intake, eliminating salt, sweating heavily and/or using diuretics.

Dumbbell – Weight used for exercising consisting of rigid handle about 14" long with sometimes detachable metal discs at each end.

Eccentric – The lowering phase of an exercise, when the muscle lengthens. For example, lowering the weight to your chest during the bench press is the eccentric, or "negative," portion of the exercise.

Energy – The capacity to do work.

Endurance – Ability of a muscle to produce force continually over a period of time.

Essential fatty acids (EFAs) – Fats our bodies can't make, so we must obtain them through our diets. These fats (which include linoleic and linolenic acid) are very important to hormone production, as well as cellular synthesis and integrity. Good sources of these fats arc flaxseed oil and safflower oil.

Estrogen – Female sex hormone.

Exercise – Each individual movement (e.g., a seated pulley row, barbell curl, or seated calf raise) that you perform in your bodybuilding workouts.

Extension – Body part (i.e. hand, neck, trunk, etc.) going from a bent to a straight position, as in leg extension.

Failure – That point in an exercise at which you have so fully fatigued your working muscles that they can no longer complete an additional repetition of a movement with strict biomechanics. You should always take your post-warm-up sets at least to the point of momentary muscular failure, and frequently past that point.

Fascia – Fibrous connective tissue that covers, supports and separates muscles and muscle groups. It also unites skin with underlying tissue.

Fast-Twitch – Refers to muscle cells that fire quickly and are utilised in anaerobic activities like sprinting and powerlifting.

Fat – One of the macronutrients. Fat contains nine calories per gram; it has the most calories of the macronutrients. There are two types of fat-saturated "bad" fat and unsaturated "good" fat.

Flex – Bend or decrease angle of a joint; contract a muscle.

Flexibility – A suppleness of joints, muscle masses, and connective tissues which lets you move your limbs over an exaggerated range of motion, a valuable quality in body-building training, since it promotes optimum physical development. Flexibility can only be attained through systematic stretching training, which should form a cornerstone of your overall bodybuilding philosophy.

Flexion – Bending in contrast to extending, as in leg flexions.

Flush – Cleanse a muscle by increasing the blood supply to it, removing toxins left in muscle by exertion.

Forced Reps – Forced reps are a frequently used method of extending a set past the point of failure to induce greater gains in muscle mass and quality. With forced reps, a training partner pulls upward on the bar just enough for you to grind out two or three reps past the failure threshold.

Form – This is simply another word to indicate the biomechanics used during the performance of any bodybuilding or weight-training movement. Perfect form involves moving only the muscles specified in an exercise description.

Free Weights – Barbells, dumbbells, and related equipment. Serious bodybuilders use a combination of free weights and such exercise machines as those manufactured by Nautilus and Universal Gyms, but they primarily use free weights in their workouts.

Fructose – The main type of sugar found in fruit. It's sweeter than sucrose (table sugar).

Giant Sets – Series of 4-6 exercises done with little or no rest between movements and a rest interval of 3-4 minutes between giant sets. You can perform giant sets for either two antagonistic muscle groups or a single body part.

Glucose – The simplest sugar molecule. It's also the main sugar found in blood and is used as a basic fuel for the body.

Gluteals – Abbreviation for gluteus maximus, medius and minimus; the buttocks muscles.

Glycogen – The principal stored form of carbohydrate energy (glucose), which is reserved in muscles. When your muscles are full of glycogen, they look and feel full.

Grazing – This term refers to frequent feedings – eating small amounts of food often.

HDL – This stands for "high-density lipoprotein." It's one of the subcategories of cholesterol – typically thought of as the "good" cholesterol. You may be able to raise your HDL cholesterol levels by ingesting quality unsaturated fats like flaxseed oil. Exercise has ~so been shown to increase HDL levels.

Hypertrophy – The scientific term denoting an increase in muscle mass and an improvement in relative muscular strength. Hypertrophy is induced by placing an "over-load" on the working muscles with various training techniques during a bodybuilding workout.

IFBB – International Federation of Bodybuilders, founded in 1946 – group that oversees worldwide men's and women's amateur and professional bodybuilding.

Intensity – The relative degree of effort that you put into each set of every exercise in a bodybuilding workout.

Isokinetic Exercise – Isotonic exercise in which there is ACCOMMODATING RESISTANCE. Also refers to constant speed. Nautilus and Cybex are two types of isokinetic machines, where machine varies amount of resistance being lifted to match force curve developed by the muscle.

Isometric Exercise – Muscular contraction where muscle maintains a constant length and joints do not move. These exercises are usually performed against a wall or other immovable object.

Isolation Exercise – In contrast to a basic exercise, an isolation movement stresses a single muscle group (or sometimes just part of a single muscle) in relative isolation from the remainder of the body. Isolation exercises are good for shaping and defining various muscle groups. For your thighs, squats would be a typical basic movement, while leg extensions would be the equivalent isolation exercise.

Isotonic Exercise – Muscular action in which there is a change in length of muscle and weight keeping tension constant. Lifting free weights is a classic isotonic exercise.

Kinesiology – Study of muscles and their movements.

Knee Wraps – Elastic strips about 3½" wide used to wrap knees for better support when performing squats, dead lifts, etc.

Lats – Abbreviation for latissimus dorsi, the large muscles of the back that move the arms downward, backward and in internal rotation.

LDL – This stands for "low-density lipoprotein" and is a subcategory of cholesterol, typically thought of as the "bad" cholesterol. Levels of LDL cholesterol can be elevated by ingestion of saturated fats and a lack of exercise.

Lean Body Mass – Everything in the body except fat, including bone, organs, skin, nails and all body tissue including muscle. Approximately 50-60% of lean body mass is water.

Ligament – Strong, fibrous band of connecting tissue connecting 2 or more bones or cartilages or supporting a muscle, fascia or organ.

Linoleic acid – An essential fatty acid and, more specifically, an omega-6 polyunsaturated fatty acid. Good sources of this fatty acid are safflower oil and soybean oil.

Linolenic acid – An essential fatty acid and, more precisely an omega-3 polyunsaturated fatty acid. It is found in high concentrations in flaxseed oil.

Lock Out – Partial repetition of an exercise by pushing the weight through only last few inches of movement.

Lower Abs – Abbreviation for abdominal muscles below the navel.

Mass – The relative size of each muscle group, or of the entire physique. As long as you also have a high degree of muscularity and good balance of physical proportions, muscle mass is a highly prized quality among competitive bodybuilders.

Max – Maximum effort for one repetition of an exercise.

Meal – Food that's eaten at one time. Each meal should contain a portion (which is the size of the palm of your hand or your clenched fist) of protein and a portion of carbohydrates.

Metabolic rate – The rate you convert energy stores into working energy in your body. In other words, it's how fast your "whole system" runs. The metabolic rate is controlled by a number of factors, including: muscle mass (the greater your muscle mass, the greater your metabolic rate), calorie intake, and exercise.

Metabolism – The use of nutrients by the body. It's the process by which substances come into the body and the rate at which they are used.

Midsection – Muscles of abdominal area, including upper and lower abdominals, obliques and rectus abdominis muscles.

Military press – Pressing a barbell from upper chest upward in standing or sitting position.

Minerals – Naturally occurring, inorganic substances that are essential for human life, which play a role in many vital metabolic processes.

Muscle – Tissue consisting of fibres organised into bands or bundles that contract to cause bodily movement.

Muscle Spasm – Sudden, involuntary contraction of muscle or muscle group.

Muscle Tone – Condition in which a muscle is in a constant yet slight state of contraction and appears firm.

Muscularity – An alternative term for "definition" or "cuts".

Myositis – Muscular soreness due to inflammation that often occurs 1-2 days after unaccustomed exercise.

Nautilus – Isokinetic type exercise machine, which attempts to match resistance with user's force.

Negative Reps – One or two partners help you lift a weight up to 50% heavier than you would normally lift to finish point of movement. Then you slowly lower weight on your own.

Nutrients – Components of food that help nourish the body: that is, they provide energy or serve as "building materials". These nutrients include carbohydrates, fats, proteins, vitamins, minerals, water, etc.

Nutrition – The applied science of eating to foster greater health, fitness, and muscular gains.

Obliques – Abbreviation for external obliques, the muscles to either side of abdominals that rotate and flex the trunk.

Olympic Barbell – A special type of barbell used in weightlifting and powerlifting competitions, but also used by bodybuilders in heavy basic exercises such as squats, bench presses, barbell bent rows, standing barbell curls, standing barbell presses, and deadlifts. An Olympic barbell sans collars weighs 45 pounds, and each collar weighs five pounds.

Olympic Lifting – The type of weightlifting competition contested at the Olympic Games every four years, as well as at national and international competitions each year. Two lifts (the snatch and the clean and jerk) are contested in a wide variety of weight classes.

Overload Principle – Applying a greater load than normal to a muscle to increase its capability.

Partial Reps – Performing an exercise without going through a complete range of motion either at the beginning or end of a rep.

Plates – The flat discs placed on the ends of barbell and dumbbell bars to increase the weight of the apparati.

Plyometric Exercise – Where muscles are loaded suddenly and stretched, then quickly contracted to produce a movement. Athletes who must jump do these, i.e. jumping off bench to ground, quickly rebounding to another bench.

Portion – The amount of carbohydrates or protein one should eat with each meal. A portion is the size of the palm of your hand or your clenched fist.

Poundage – The amount of weight that you use in an exercise, whether that weight is on a barbell, dumbbell, or exercise machine.

Power – Strength + Speed.

Power Lifts – Three movements used in powerlifting competition: the squat, bench press and dead lift.

Power Lifting – A second form of competitive weightlifting (not contested in the Olympics, however) featuring three lifts: the squat, bench press, and dead lift. Power lifting is contested both nationally and internationally in a wide variety of weight classes for both men and women.

Power Training – System of weight training using low repetitions, heavy weights.

Progression – The act of gradually adding to the amount of resistance that you use in each exercise. Without consistent progression in your workouts, you won't overload your muscles sufficiently to promote optimum increases in hypertrophy.

Progressive Resistance – Method of training where weight is increased as muscles gain strength and endurance, the backbone of all weight training.

Proteins – Proteins are the building blocks of muscle, enzymes, and sonic hormones. They are made up of amino acids and are essential for growth and repair in the body. A gram of protein contains four calories. Those from animal sources contain the essential amino acids. Those from vegetable sources contain some but not all of the essential amino acids. Proteins are broken up by the body to produce amino acids.

Pump – The tight, blood-congested feeling in a muscle after it has been intensely trained. Muscle pump is caused by a rapid influx of blood into the muscles to remove fatigue toxins and replace supplies of fuel and oxygen. A good muscle pump indicates that you have optimally worked a muscle group.

Pumped – Slang meaning the muscles have been made large by increasing blood supply to them through exercise.

Pumping Iron – Phrase that has been in use since the 1950s, but recently greatly popularised. Lifting weights.

Quads – Abbreviation for quadriceps femoris muscles, muscles on top of legs, which consist of 4 parts (heads).

Quality Training – Training just before bodybuilding competition where intervals between sets are drastically reduced to enhance muscle mass and density, and low-calorie diet is followed to reduce body fat.

Repetition (rep) – The number of times you lift and lower a weight in one set of an exercise. For example, if you lift and lower a weight 10 times before setting the weight down, you have completed 10 "reps" in one set.

Reps – Abbreviation for REPETITIONS.

Resistance exercise – Working out with weights or using your body to resist some other force. This includes a wide spectrum of motion, from push-ups to dumbbell curls.

Rest Pause Training – Training method where you press out one difficult repetition, then replace bar in stands, then after a 10-20 second rest, do another rep, etc.

Rest period – The amount of time you allow between sets and exercises.

Ripped – Slang meaning extreme muscularity.

Routine – Also called a training schedule or programme, a routine is the total list of exercises, sets, and reps (and sometimes weights) used in one training session.

Set – Group of reps (lifting and lowering a weight) of an exercise after which you take a brief rest period. For example, if you complete 10 reps, set the weight down, complete eight more reps, set the weight down again, and repeat for six more reps, you have completed three sets of the exercise.

Sleeve – The hollow metal tube that fits over the bar on most exercise barbell and dumbbell sets. This sleeve makes it easier for the bar to rotate in your hands as you do an exercise.

Spotters – Training partners who stand by to act as safety helpers when you perform such heavy exercises as squats and bench presses. If you get stuck under the weight or begin to lose control of it, spotters can rescue you and prevent needless injuries.

Slow-Twitch – Muscle cells that contract slowly, are resistant to fatigue and are utilised in endurance activities such as long-distance running, cycling or swimming.

Snatch – Olympic lift where weight is lifted from floor to overhead, (with arms extended) in one continuous movement (see also CLEAN AND JERK).

Spot – Assist if called upon by someone performing an exercise.

Spotter – Person who watches a partner closely to see if any help is needed during a specific exercise.

Sticking Point – A stalling out of bodybuilding progress.

Straight Sets – Groups of repetitions (SETS) interrupted by only brief pauses (30-90 seconds).

Strength – The ability of a muscle to produce maximum amount of force.

Strength Training – Using resistance weight training to build maximum muscle force.

Stretching – A type of exercise programme in which you assume exaggerated postures that stretch muscles, joints, and connective tissues, hold these positions for several seconds, relax and then repeat the postures. Regular stretching exercise promotes body flexibility.

Striations – Grooves or ridge marks seen under the skin, the ultimate degree of muscle definition.

Super Set – Alternating back and forth between two exercises until the prescribed number of sets is complete.

Supplement – This is a term used to describe a preparation such as a tablet, pill, or powder that contains nutrients. Supplements are used to help you achieve optimal nutrient intake.

Symmetry – The shape or general outline of a person's body, as when seen in silhouette. If you have good symmetry, you will have relatively wide shoulders, flaring lats, a small waist-hip structure, and generally small joints.

Tendon – A band or cord of strong, fibrous tissue that connects muscles to bone.

Testosterone – The male hormone primarily responsible for the maintenance of muscle mass and strength induced by heavy training. Testosterone is secondarily responsible for developing such secondary male sex characteristics as a deep voice, body hair, and male pattern baldness.

Tone – See MUSCLE TONE.

Training Straps – Also known as lifting straps. Cotton or leather straps wrapped around wrists, then under and over a bar held by clenched hands to aid in certain lifts (rowing, chin-ups, shrugs, dead lifts, cleans, etc.) where you might lose your grip before working muscle to desired capacity.

Training to Failure – Continuing a set until it is impossible to compete another rep without assistance.

Traps – Abbreviation for trapezius muscles, the largest muscles of the back and neck that draw head backward and rotate scapula.

Trimming Down – To gain hard muscular appearance by losing body fat.

Tri Sets – Alternating back and forth between 3 exercises until prescribed number of sets is completed.

Universal Law of Reciprocation – The more you help others, the more your life is enhanced.

Unsaturated fat – These are "good" fats. They are called unsaturated because they have one or more open spots on their carbon skeletons. This category of fats includes the essential fatty acids linoleic and linolenic. The main sources of these fats are from plant foods, such as safflower, sunflower, and flaxseed oils.

Upper Abs – Abbreviation for abdominal muscles above navel.

Variable Resistance – Strength training equipment where the machine varies amount of weight being lifted to match strength curve for a particular exercise, usually with a cam, lever arm or hydraulic cylinder. Also referred to as "ACCOMMODATING RESISTANCE."

Vascularity – Increase in size and number of observable veins. Highly desirable in bodybuilding.

Vitamins – Organic compounds that are vital to life, indispensable to bodily function, and needed in minute amounts. They are calorie-free essential nutrients. Many of them function as coenzymes, supporting a multitude of biological functions.

Warm-up – The 10-15-minute session of light calisthenics, aerobic exercise, and stretching taken prior to handling heavy bodybuilding training movements. A good warm-up helps to prevent injuries and actually allows you to get more out of your training than if you went into a workout totally cold.

Weight – The same as Poundage or Resistance.

Weightlifting – The competitive form of weight training in which each athlete attempts to lift as much as he can in well-defined exercises. Olympic lifting and power lifting are the two types of weightlifting competition.

Weight Training Belt – Thick leather belt used to support lower back. Used while doing squats, military presses, dead lifts, bent rowing, etc.

Workout – A bodybuilding or weight-training session.